Diagnostic Cystoscopy

Bradley C. Tenny • Michael O'Neill

Diagnostic Cystoscopy

The Cystoscopist Reference

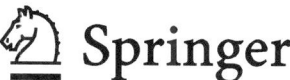 Springer

Bradley C. Tenny
Atrium Health Urology Department
Charlotte, NC, USA

Michael O'Neill
Atrium Health Urology Department
Charlotte, NC, USA

ISBN 978-3-031-10667-5   ISBN 978-3-031-10668-2   (eBook)
https://doi.org/10.1007/978-3-031-10668-2

This Springer imprint is published by the registered company Springer Nature Switzerland AG
The registered company address is: Gewerbestrasse 11, 6330 Cham, Switzerland

Remember to take pride in developing mastery over an important urologic procedure. Endoscopy has been performed since the 1800s; with each novel adaptation providing better visualization and the ability to better people's lives. Remember that we stand on the shoulders of giants who came before us.

Preface

Diagnostic cystoscopy is the gold standard procedure in assessing anatomical variations and/or bladder pathologies. For example, for a clinician to adequately rule out urothelial cancer of the bladder the clinician must directly visualize the whole bladder. Mastering this skill is thus incredibly important for training MD and advanced practice provider (Nurse Practitioner or Physician Assistant), and once mastered a readily available reference would serve to benefit the said clinician in differentiating benign and malignant pathologies.

This textbook is written as a comprehensive review by experts in the field of Urology on cystoscope, including both the flexible and rigid instrument, technical use, and certainly bladder pathologies. Thus, being remarkably familiar with these instruments is vital in being a great cystoscopist.

Lastly and most significantly, this book covers numerous topics in normal anatomy, benign and malignant urethral pathology, and benign and malignant bladder pathology. Dialog on each presented topic includes a brief pathological discussion, associated clinical significance such as common signs or symptoms, the suggested treatment for said topic, additional references for further reading, and importantly photographs. Photographs are included on every topic, with a minimum of one image and a maximum of five for reference. If this book is well received, possible future editions will serve to add additional photos and discuss pediatric topics in more refined detail.

Availability of a comprehensive reference on diagnostic cystoscopy has been needed for quite some time, and this book satisfies this need, both for the developing and experienced cystoscopist.

Charlotte, NC, USA   Bradley C. Tenny, MSN, AGACNP, CUNP
Charlotte, NC, USA   Michael O'Neill, MD, FACS

Contents

Chapter 1
Introduction to Cystoscopy

1.1 Parts of the Cystoscope

1.1.1 Rigid Cystourethroscope

A rigid cystoscope is made up of three parts: The outer sheath, the lens/scope, and lastly the bridge otherwise explained as the working channel (see Fig. 1.1). There are a few manufactures that make the rigid cystoscope including Olympus, Karl Storz, Gyrus/ACMI, and Wolf. The picture of the rigid cystoscope in this book pertains to the Olympus cystoscope. Sheath sizes vary in French size and have accommodating obturators for blind introduction into the bladder. Bridges can be either single-channel or multi-channel.

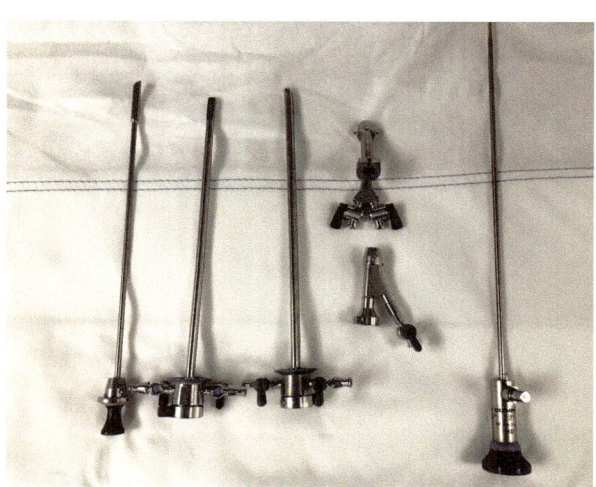

Fig. 1.1 Rigid cystoscope broken up

© The Author(s), under exclusive license to Springer Nature
Switzerland AG 2022
B. C. Tenny, M. O'Neill, *Diagnostic Cystoscopy*,
https://doi.org/10.1007/978-3-031-10668-2_1

Photos of the rigid cystoscope are few given that this book's purpose is to educate the clinician on diagnostic cystoscopy, typically performed with a flexible scope in the office. Again, diagnostic cystoscopy is performed whenever a camera is placed within the bladder, thus understanding of the rigid instrument is additionally important.

1.1.2 Flexible Cystourethroscope

Flexible scopes allow for complete assessment of the bladder's superficial lining, the mucosa. Flexible cameras are what is commonly employed for diagnostic cystoscopies. These cameras range in size between 16 and 17 French and are additionally manufactured by the aforementioned companies. The scopes have a single working chamber for both irrigation and the passage of instruments (see Fig. 1.2). When performing a task, such as a biopsy, irrigation should also be running to allow for adequate visualization. The use of a three-way valve allows for continued flow while passage of an instrument through a diaphragm to ensure no leakage of irrigation (see Figs. 1.3 and 1.4).

Flexible cystourethroscopes come in a few options. Scopes can be either be fiberoptic/analog or digital. Digital scopes can come in both standard and high definition (See Figs. 1.5 and 1.6). Digital scopes do not require focusing or white balancing prior to instrumentation. In short, digital scopes typically have a higher degree of resolution.

Fig. 1.2 Digital flexible cystoscope

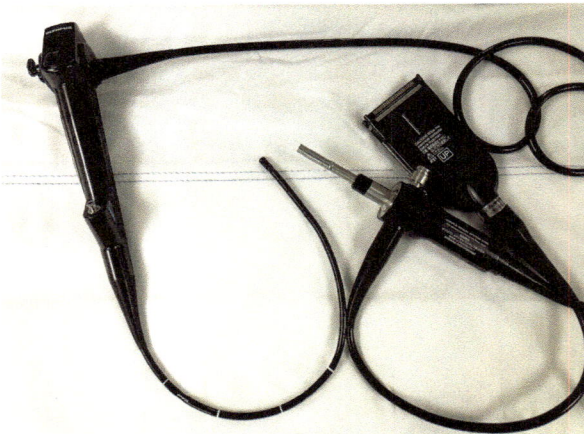

Fig. 1.3 Three-way valve with stopper diaphragm

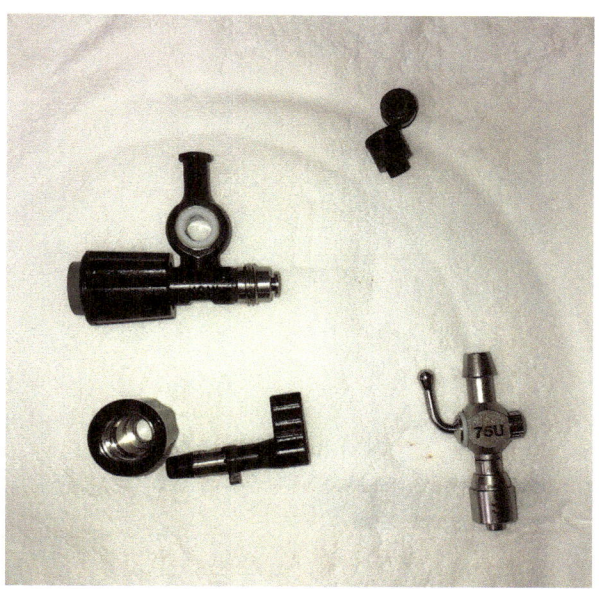

Fig. 1.4 Flexible grasper for the rigid cystoscope

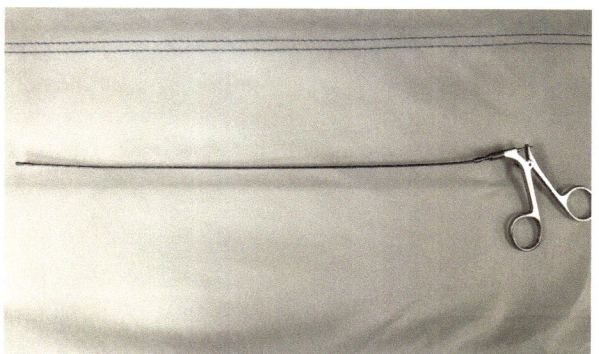

Fig. 1.5 Light cord for analog cystoscope

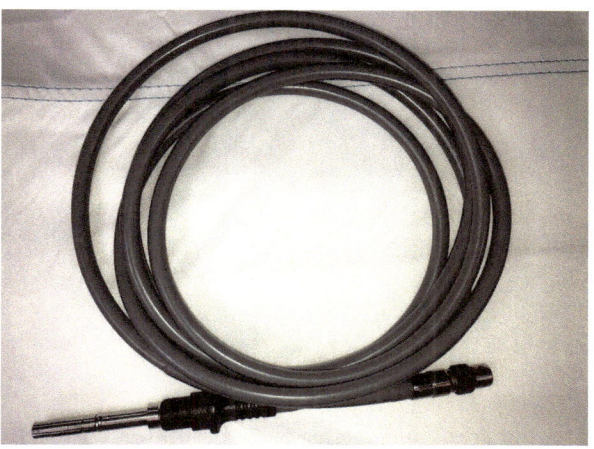

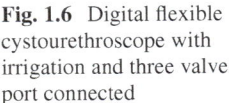

Fig. 1.6 Digital flexible cystourethroscope with irrigation and three valve port connected

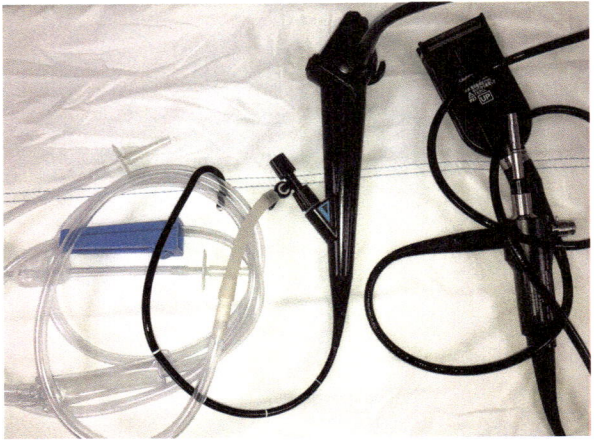

1.2 Operative Technique

1.2.1 Positioning

First, it is imperative to position the patient so that he or she is comfortable and to allow for ease of performance/scope passage by the clinician. The preferred positions are supine for a flexible cystoscope or lithotomy for a rigid cystoscope. After the patient has been adequately positioned the clinician should prep the patient using either betadine or chlorhexidine-soaked gauze or swabs.

1.2.2 Physical Exam

Next, prior to the introduction of any scope within the urethra the clinician must perform a physical exam. Is important to pay close attention for any cutaneous lesions or anatomic abnormalities that may make the procedure difficult. For instance, the recognition of meatal stenosis would require meatal dilation prior to the introduction of a 16 French flexible scope.

1.2.3 Passage of the Scope

In men, the penis should be placed on complete traction or stretch at the angulation of 90 to 45 degrees towards the patient's feet. If performing cystoscopy using the rigid scope, it is best to hold the penis at the 90 degrees for introduction with lowering of the penis and the scope simultaneously as the scope reaches the membranous urethra prior to the prostatic urethra. With the flexible scope again, the penis is held on stretch with clinician's nondominant hand between the ring and middle finger. With the dominant hand, the scope is brought closer to the patient's penis and the tip of the scope is guided into the urethral meatus using the index and thumb finger. The scope is only inserted after adequate lubrication and after the irrigation has been turned on. If an assistant is present, he or she may hold the scope while the clinician directs the flexible cystoscope into the urethral meatus using both hands. This is very helpful in patients who may have a large body habitus. Once the scope has been inserted in the urethra, the clinician should grab the scope with the dominant hand ensuring that the scope does not retract out of the penis requiring the procedure to be repeated; introduction of the instrument is often the most reported anxiety producing part, it is important to only to have to do this once.

After having passed the scope through the anterior urethra, with the penis remaining on stretch, the clinician will reach the membranous urethra. The scope is then directed anteriorly using a small degree of flexion in order to transverse the external genitourinary diaphragm. With further advancement of the scope, the clinician readily reaches the prostatic urethra. At this point the scope should nearly be fully flexed, in similar fashion to the tip of a coudé catheter, in order to gain access to the bladder neck and the bladder.

In women, the clinician retracts both the labia majora and minora exposing the vulvar vestibule. With advancement of the scope using the contralateral hand the index and thumb guide the scope into the urethral meatus (see Fig. 1.7). The female urethra is on average only 2–3 cm and access grants near immediate entrance into the bladder (see Figs. 1.8 and 1.9). In certain situations, it may be easier having an assistant hold the scope with passage into the urethra for either female or male.

Fig. 1.7 Passage of the cystoscope into the female urethra meatus

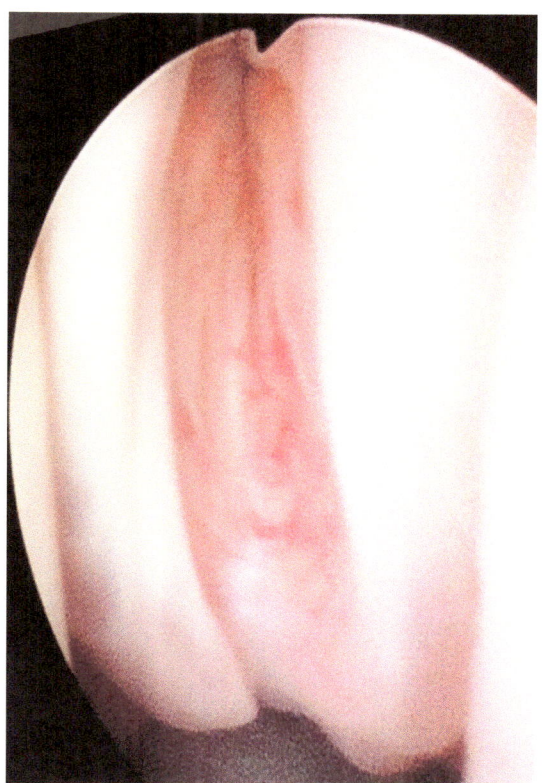

Fig. 1.8 Passage of the cystoscope into the female urethra, continued

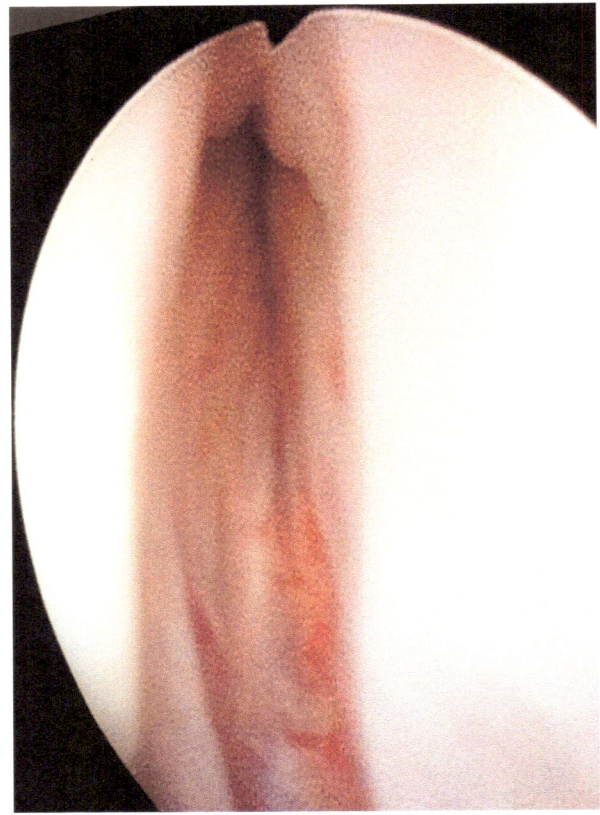

Fig. 1.9 Cystoscopic assessment of the female genitourinary diaphragm/internal sphincter

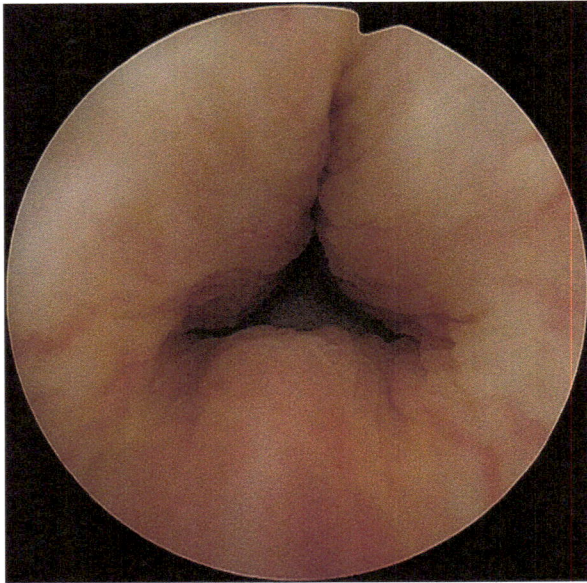

Upon entrance into the bladder, the clinician performs systematic evaluation (see Fig. 1.10). Irrigation could either be running maximally or turned off if the bladder is noted to have small compliance or already be full of urine. If visualization is impaired by hematuria or any other opaque fluid, the clinician may turn off the irrigation and disconnect the three-valve allowing for the bladder to empty through the scope. If this is considered, it would best be performed in a patient who is sedated, as this will prolong the procedure.

Fig. 1.10 Female bladder neck with visualization of the bladder lumen

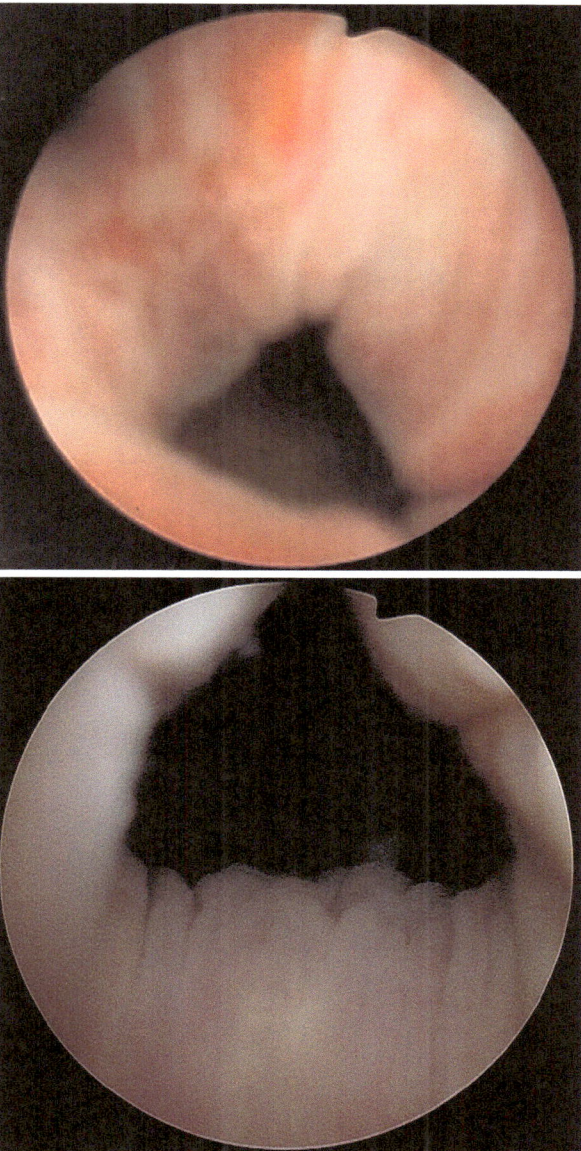

Systematic evaluation of the bladder typically involves initial assessment of the trigone and the posterior wall of the bladder (see Fig. 1.11). The number, location, and appearance of ureteral orifices should be characterized. The clinician should wait for reflux from either ureter to ensure no obstruction and/or bloody urine output. Visualization of the bladder's lateral walls is performed by rotating the cystoscope while keeping the camera orientation fixed. The dome and anterior wall of the bladder are identified by localization of an air bubble due to introduction of the scope. The procedure is completed after retroflexion in order to assess the bladder neck (see Fig. 1.12). Rotation of the scope while remaining fully flexed allows for a complete circumferential assessment of the bladder neck.

Fig. 1.11 Access into the bladder's lumen

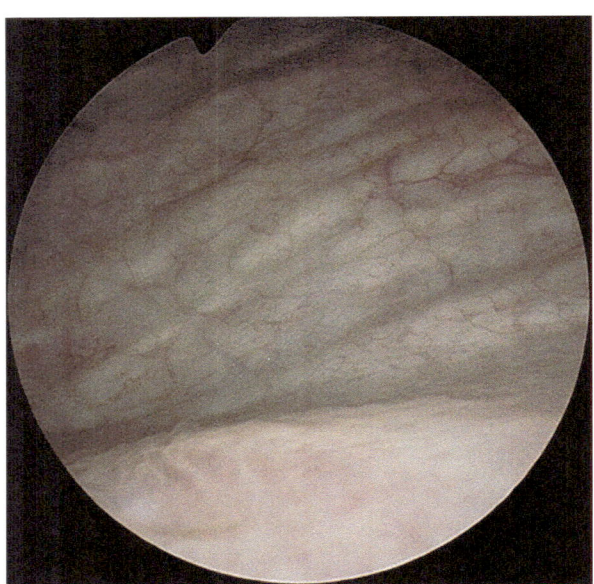

Fig. 1.12 Retroflexion assessment of the bladder neck in a female urethra

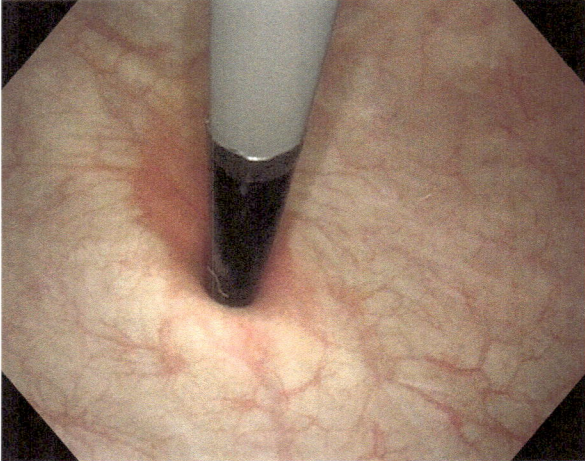

Stepwise Approach to Diagnostic Cystoscopy
1. Men—Grasp penis in nondominant hand, hold on stretch at 45–90 degrees, while simultaneously holding the scope in the dominant hand.

    Women—With nondominant hand retract labia to expose urethral meatus, with dominant hand holding scope bring scope towards vulvar vestibule advancing the tip of scope toward the retracting hand.
2. Using the index finger and thumb of the nondominant hand providing exposure advance tip of scope into urethral meatus.
3. Gently lower/advance scope further into the urethra.

    Men—Continue advancing the scope into the pendulous urethra until the bulbar urethra is reached. Once the bulbar urethra is reached, begin flexing the scope anterior toward the urogenital diaphragm in order to access the prostatic urethra and the bladder neck.

    Women—The urethra should be assessed in its entirety; it is much easier upon scope withdrawal as the female urethra is only 2-3 cm on average.
4. Advance scope into the bladder. Upon access into the bladder, wait a few seconds to allow for some distention if decompressed.
5. Upon entrance into the bladder assess the bladder's base, trigone ridge, and posterior wall. With assessment of the trigone ridge, rotate your dominant hand to rotate the scope following the ridge to the ureteral orifice.
6. Assess both ureteral orifices to ensure normal efflux.
7. Assess the lateral walls, starting systematically from the lower anterior corner to the superior edge. It does not matter what side you start with.
8. Assess the bladder's anterior wall by identification of the bubble lying superiorly in the supine patient. Be sure to not allow the bubble to obscure any mucosal lesion.
9. Assess bladder neck, by fully flexing the scope performing retroflexion. Rotate your wrist in a supination and pronation fashion to circumferentially assess the bladder neck.
10. Release flexion and slowly retract the scope out of the bladder assessing the bladder neck and urethra once more on the way out.

1.3   Clinical Pearls

1.3.1   Indications for Diagnostic Cystoscopy

1. Hematuria, gross or microscopic.
2. Known or previously identified malignancy of the urethra or the bladder.
3. Lower urinary tract symptoms/voiding dysfunction.
4. Trauma.
5. Possible removal of foreign bodies.

1.3.2   Pre-procedural Considerations

1.3.2.1   Consent and Preop Urine Assessment

Prior to performing any invasive procedure, informed consent should be obtained by the patient with a nurse witness. A urinalysis or urine culture is indicated if there are risk factors involving the patient. The AUA and the European Association of Urology have published recommendations regarding periprocedural antibiotics [1], and they are worth the review. Please see the reference section for the AUA's respective article. In short explanation, however, neither organization recommends antimicrobial prophylaxis for routine diagnostic cystoscopy. Risk factors that would predispose the patient to infection warranting periprocedural antimicrobial therapy include: advanced age, anatomic anomalies with urinary tract, poor nutritional status, smoking, chronic corticosteroid use, immunodeficiency, externalized catheters, colonized endogenous or exogenous material, distant coexistent infection, and prolonged hospitalization. Traditionally, antibiotic prophylaxis consists of administration of a one-time dose of fluoroquinolone, trimethoprim combination med, and/or first-generation cephalosporin. Duration of procedural antibiotics should not exceed 24 h, unless indicated by an evolving illness.

1.3.2.2   Decreasing Pain

The ample use of lubrication, ensuring continuous flow of irrigation while passing the instrument, and not accidentally retracting the scope back into the urethra requiring reinsertion are the main techniques that any clinician can do to decrease pain. Certain facilities may have lidocaine infused gel; a topical anesthetic gel could be an option; however, literature has not always demonstrated a therapeutic effect [2]. It likely depends on the length of the procedure, the length of dwell time of the anesthetic, and the amount of lubrication. Lastly, there is literature demonstrating that allowing the patient to visualize the procedure causes a reduction in reported pain [3].

1.3.3   Complications of Diagnostic Cystoscopy

Complications of diagnostic cystoscopy are rare, and the procedure is typically well tolerated [4]. Nonetheless, the risk of significant infection should always be considered in patients with predisposing risk factors, such as, advanced age, anatomic anomalies with urinary tract, poor nutritional status, smoking, chronic corticosteroid use, immunodeficiency, externalized catheters, colonized endogenous or exogenous material, distant coexistent infection, and prolonged hospitalization. Antimicrobial prophylaxis is warranted for instrumentation in these patient populations. Research or literature demonstrating the risk of urinary tract infection again is limited in the ambulatory patient population. In a study of 3108 patient cystoscopies without antibiotic prophylaxis, 673 had asymptomatic bacteriuria and 2435 had sterile urine, afebrile urinary tract infection occurred in only 59 patients within 30 days of cystoscopy: equaling an incidence of 1.9% [5].

1.4   Innovations in the Field

A relatively recent innovation in diagnostic cystoscopy is use of a blue light, commonly known as blue light cystoscopy (see Fig. 1.13). Blue light cystoscopy involves the installation of a photosensitizer into the bladder prior to introduction of the scope via the use of a catheter. The photosensitizers then induce accumulation of protoporphyrins in any rapidly dividing/mitotic cell, such as occurs in malignant cells. The protoporphyrins are then converted into the photoactive porphyrins, which then fluoresce red when illuminated using a blue light [6].

There have been numerous studies that have documented the improved tumor detection rates using blue light cystoscopy. For instance, systemic reviews reveal a 7 to 29% increase in the rate of small papillary tumors identified using blue light cystoscopy over standard white light cystoscopy [7].

Narrow band imaging is another technique to enhance detection of malignant lesions (see Fig. 1.14). Narrow band imaging light is two specific wavelengths of light that are taken up by hemoglobin, versus white light being the "complete spectrum." This appears with increased/improved visualizations of blood vessels or blood. Cancers are known to induce angiogenesis, and thus appear prominent with this technique (see Fig. 1.15). Past research has demonstrated increased tumor detection rates [8].

Lastly, disposable flexible cystoscopes are a recent innovation that offer the possibility of increased procedures performed by a clinician per day, as these instruments do not need to be sterilized between patients (see Fig. 1.16). As this innovation is new, further research may additionally yield a positive benefit in patients with multidrug-resistant colonized urologic tracts, but we must wait to see.

Bladder images under white and blue light

Standard White Light
Cystoscopy

Blue Light Cystoscopy
with Cysview

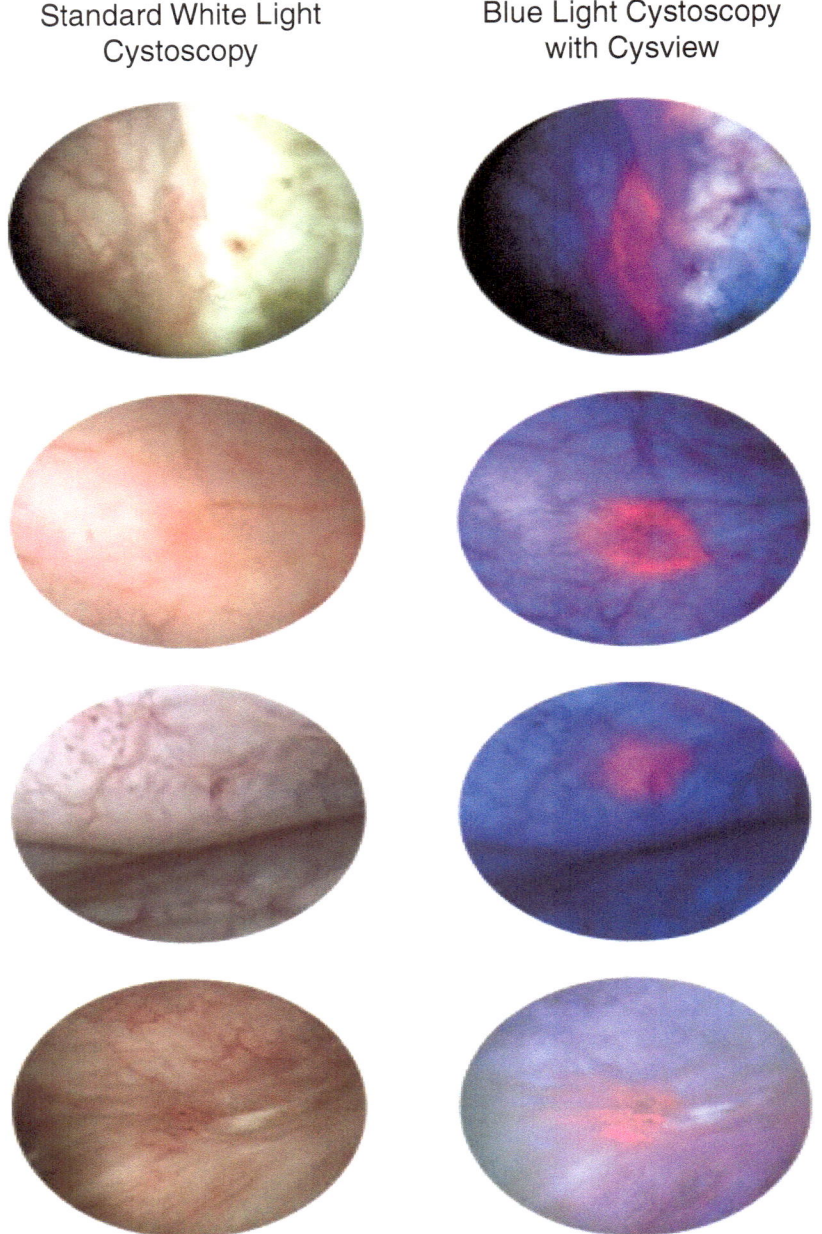

Fig. 1.13 Blue light cystoscopy comparison using Cysview/Hexvix from Photocure. Blue light cystoscopy is available and widespread in large parts of the world and are included in all the major guidelines at this stage [9]

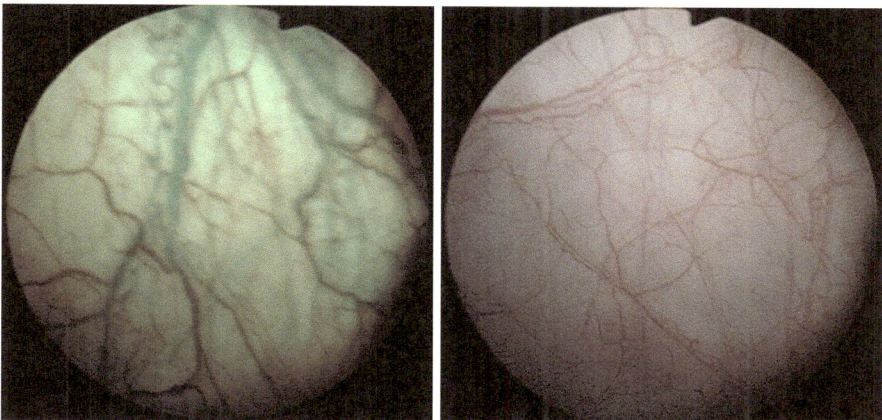

Fig. 1.14 Comparison of bladder mucosal appearance under narrow band imaging versus normal white light cystoscopy

Fig. 1.15 Papillary bladder tumor visualized under narrow band imaging

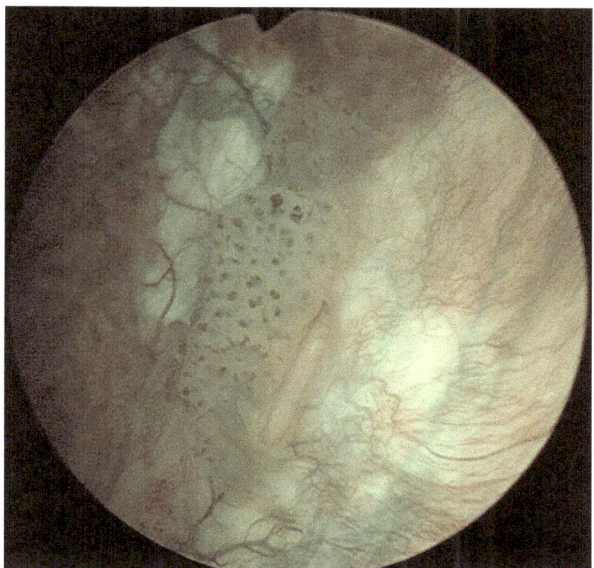

Fig. 1.16 Disposable flexible cystoscope, Ambu cysto by InnoMedicus [10]

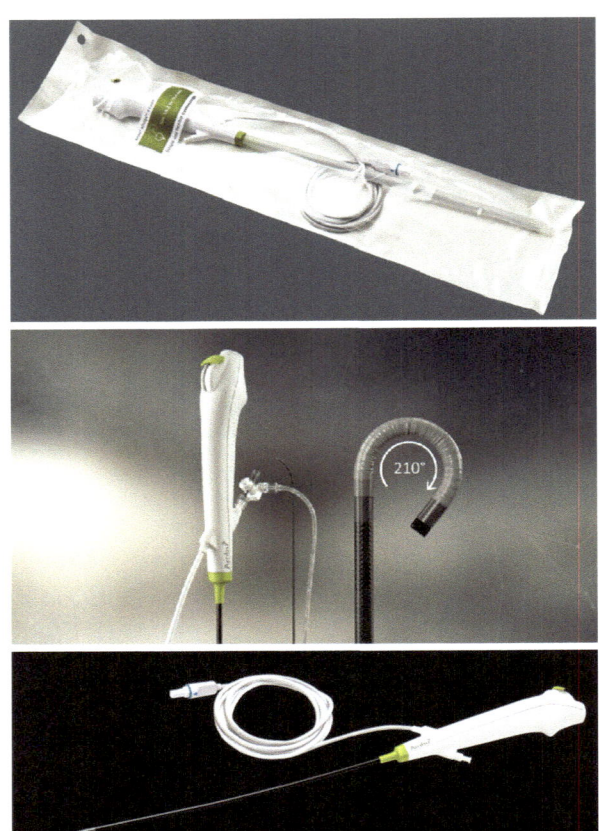

References

1. Lightner DJ, et al. Best practice statement on urologic procedures and antimicrobial prophylaxis. J Urol. 2020;256:351–6.
2. McFarlane N, Denstedt J, Ganapathy S, Razvi H. Randomized trial of 10ml and 20ml of 2% Intraurethral lidocaine gel placebo in men undergoing flexible cystoscopy. J Endourol. 2004;15(5):541–4.
3. Soomro KQ, Nasir AR, Ather MH. The impact of Patient's self-viewing of flexible cystoscopy on pain using a visual analog scale in a randmomized control trial. Urology. 2011;77:21–3.
4. Stav K, Leibovici G, Livshitz S, Linder A, Zisman A. Adverse effects of cystoscopy and its impact on Patient's quality of life and sexual performance. Isr Med Assoc J. 2004;6:474–8.
5. Garcia-Perdomo H, Lopez H, Carbonell J, al, e. Efficacy of antibiotic prophylaxis in patients undergoing cystoscopy: a randomized clinical trial. World J Urol. 2013;31:1433.
6. Zabell J, Konety B. Enhanced Cystoscopic techniques: fluorescence cystoscopy, narrow band imaging, optical coherent tomography, and confocal laser Endomicroscopy. In: Campbell-Walsh-Wein urology. Philadelphia: Elsevier; 2021. p. 3091–111.
7. Burger M, Grossman H, Droller M, Schmidbauer J, Hermann G, Dagoescu O, et al. Photodynamic diagnosis of non-muscle-invasive bladder cancer with Hexaminolevulinate

cystoscopy: a meta-analysis of detection and recurrence based on raw data. Eur Urol. 2013;64:846–54.

8. Herr H, Donat S. A comparison of white-light cystoscopy and narrow-band imaging cystoscopy to detect bladder tumour recurrences. BJU Int. 2008;102:1111–4.
9. Figure: Blue light cystoscopy comparison image using Cysview/Hexvix provided by Photocure.
10. Figure: Disposable flexible cystoscope, Ambu cysto, provided by InnoMedicus.

Chapter 2
Normal Anatomy

2.1 Male Urethra

2.1.1 Descriptive Anatomy

The urethra is the entrance to the bladder. It differs widely between sexes; it is arguably the most distinctly different anatomical body part that occurs in all sexes. The male urethra is on average 17.5 cm–20 cm long. It is divided between two distinct regions, the anterior and posterior urethra. The area that divides these two respective halves is the location of the external striated urethral sphincter or the urogenital diaphragm [1].

The anterior urethra includes the following: the urethral meatus, the fossa navicularis, the pendulous urethra/penile urethra, and the bulbar urethra. The pendulous urethra is the longest portion of the anterior urethra. The bulbar urethra is around the location of the base on the external penis (begins at the level of the suspensory ligament of the penis) and has a larger luminal caliber. The anterior urethral caliber increases as the scope gets closer to the bladder.

The posterior urethra is the remaining portion of the urethra, extending from the external striated sphincter towards the bladder neck. The first segment of the posterior urethra is called the membranous urethra. It is the shortest segment of the urethra and the least distensible. This is due to it being surrounded by the striated muscle fibers of the external urethral sphincter. The remaining parts of the posterior urethra include the prostatic urethra and the bladder neck.

The prostatic urethra includes the portion of the urethra encased by the prostate gland. This area again, is situated between the membranous urethra and the bladder neck. The whole prostate gland is shaped similar to an inverted cone, with the apex at the distal location along the urethra and the base supporting the bladder. The apex is marked internally by a urethral projection termed the verumontanum or shortened to "veru."

© The Author(s), under exclusive license to Springer Nature Switzerland AG 2022
B. C. Tenny, M. O'Neill, *Diagnostic Cystoscopy*,
https://doi.org/10.1007/978-3-031-10668-2_2

The prostate is an important accessory gland of the male reproductive system. Dr. McNeal, a scientist who vastly contributed to our understanding of prostate anatomy divides the gland into three zones: peripheral, central, and transitional. The peripheral zone of the prostate is the outer inferior portion of the gland that wraps approx. 260 degrees around the central and transitional zones conically, reminiscent of a thick incomplete ring. The peripheral zone makes up approx. 75% of the total gland's volume. The central zone encases the inferior portion of the prostatic urethra, and the transitional zone encases the lateral and superior portion of the prostatic urethra [2].

2.1.2 Cystoscopic Anatomy

Recognition of different urethral sections during cystourethroscopy is made by visible landmarks, change in urethral lumen caliber, and the trajectory of the lumen. Upon introduction of the cystoscope through the urethral meatus, the clinician arrives at the fossa navicularis. This section is dilated slightly in comparison to the pendulous/penile urethra extending proximally, which is a common location of stricture disease.

The pendulous urethral mucosa should appear flat, yellow/white with a pink tinge, and the lumen without any abrupt change in caliber (see Fig. 2.1). At the junction of the bulbar urethra the clinician should appreciate the change in mucosa to a slight increase in pink/red with an increase in caliber (see Figs. 2.2 and 2.3). The urethral lumen then takes a slight oblique trajectory superiorly where the external

Fig. 2.1 Pendulous urethra with a dangler suture for DJ stent removal. (Patient 1)

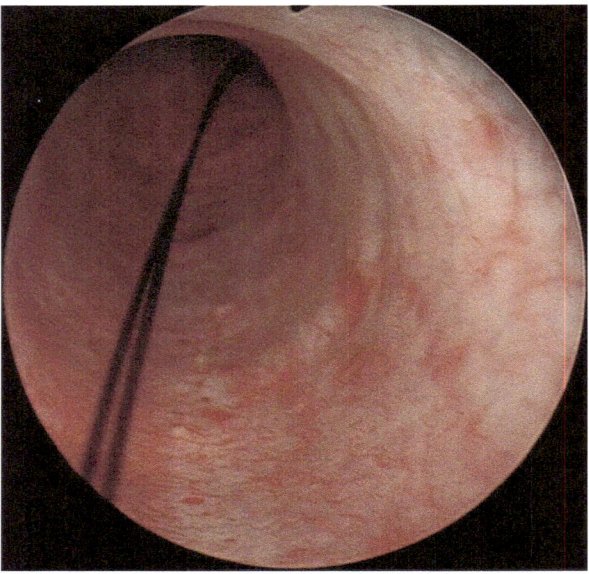

Fig. 2.2 Bulbar urethra, with the same dangler suture attached to the DJ stent is seen traversing the genitourinary sphincter positioned anterior through the slit. (Patient 1)

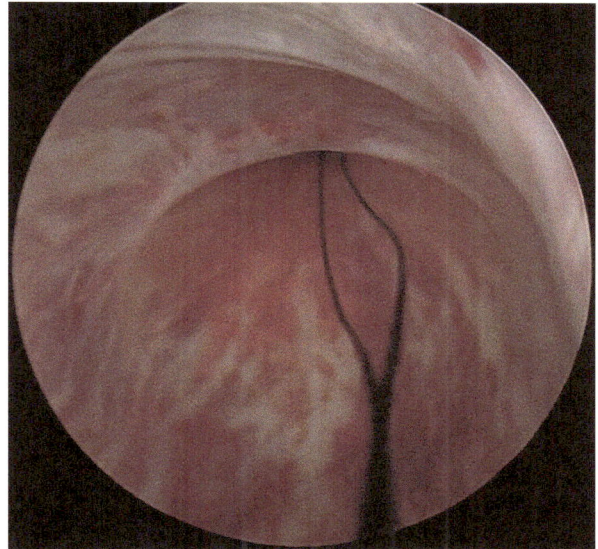

Fig. 2.3 Traversing the bulbar urethra. Notice the anterior descent of the lumen towards the sphincter and the prostatic urethra. (Patient 2)

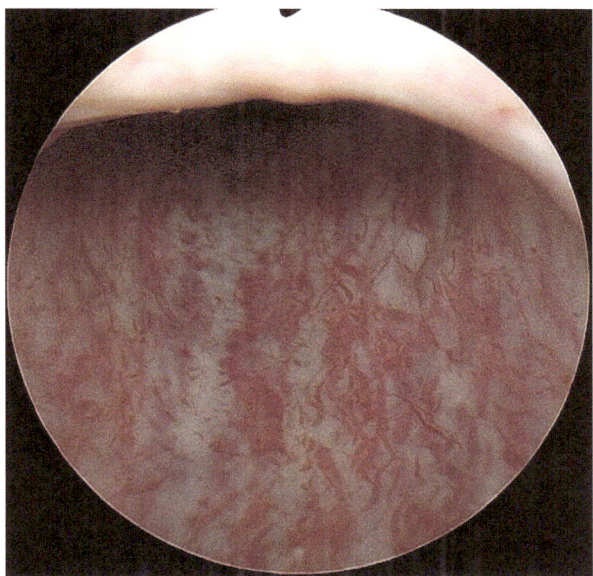

sphincter can be appreciated (see Figs. 2.4 and 2.5). The sphincter can appear with complete coaptation; however, with irrigation running on maximum it typically appears as a continued small tract (see Fig. 2.6). As previously instructed in the first chapter, to account for the oblique trajectory in urethral route, the clinician has to lower his hands in order to raise the tip of the scope.

Fig. 2.4 The bulbar urethra with the external sphincter in view. (Patient 2)

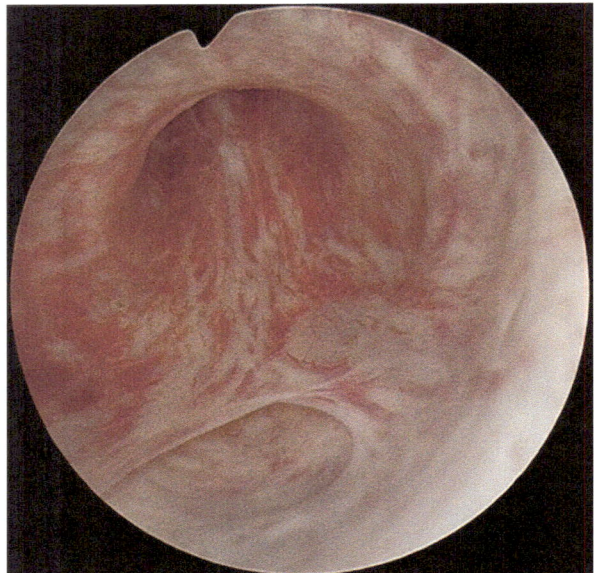

Fig. 2.5 Entering the genitourinary diaphragm/external urinary sphincter. A dangler suture is again visualized in this patient. (Patient 1)

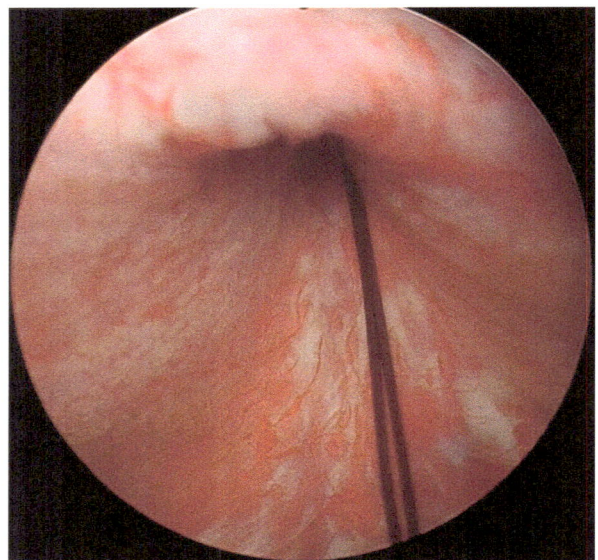

The prostatic urethra is encountered just beyond the external sphincter and is normally the largest caliber encountered upon urethroscopy. The area is marked by the veru, urethral projection, that extends a few millimeters into the urethral lumen from 6 o'clock (see Figs. 2.7 and 2.8). The veru contains the prostatic utricle and the

Fig. 2.6 The genitourinary diaphragm/external urinary sphincter at the proximal end of the bulbar urethra in the male patient. (Patient 3)

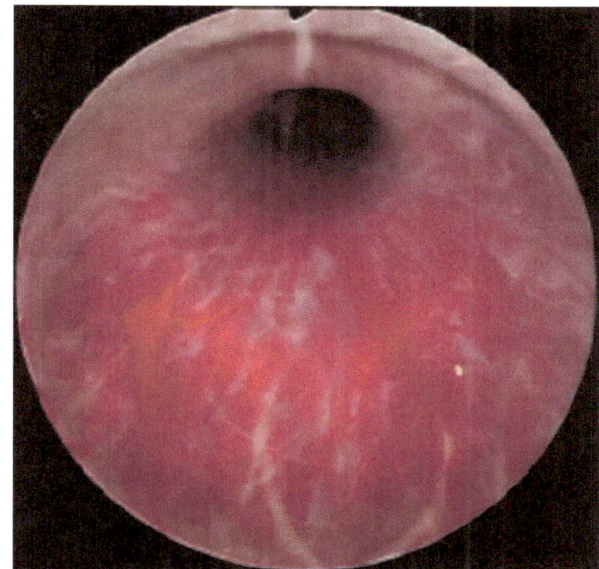

Fig. 2.7 Having crossed the genitourinary diaphragm, the prostatic urethra is approached. The prostatic urethra is demarcated by the location of the "veru" (see within the center of the above photograph). (Patient 2)

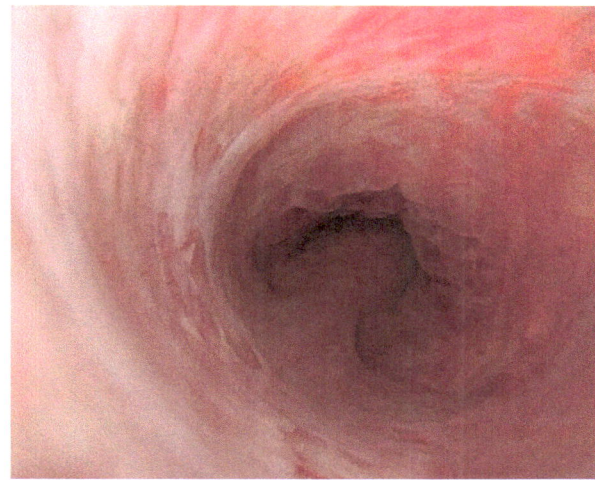

ejaculatory ducts. This is an especially important landmark to cystoscopists when performing transurethral resections of the prostate, as unintentional incision distal to this location may cause incontinence (marks the apical end of the prostate and thus external striated sphincter) (see Figs. 2.9, 2.10, and 2.11).

The bladder neck is the last area encountered prior to entering the bladder's lumen. Discussion on the cystoscopic anatomy is held within the bladder section, the following section (see Figs. 2.12 and 2.13).

Fig. 2.8 Approaching the veru/the apex of the prostatic urethra

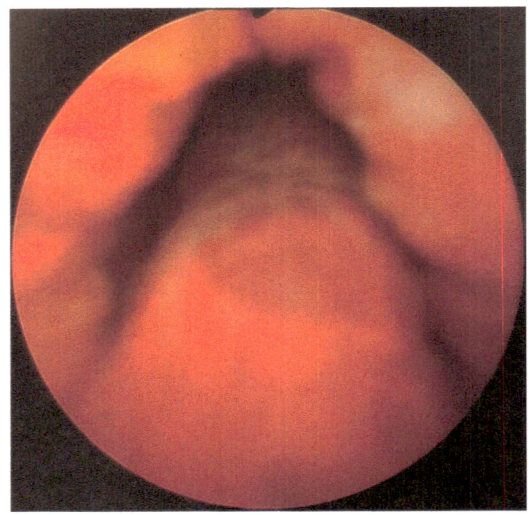

Fig. 2.9 The length of the veru is variable between patients. The above photograph demonstrates a prominent veru extending up towards the bladder neck. The below photograph pictures a small veru with no prostatic lobe hypertrophy

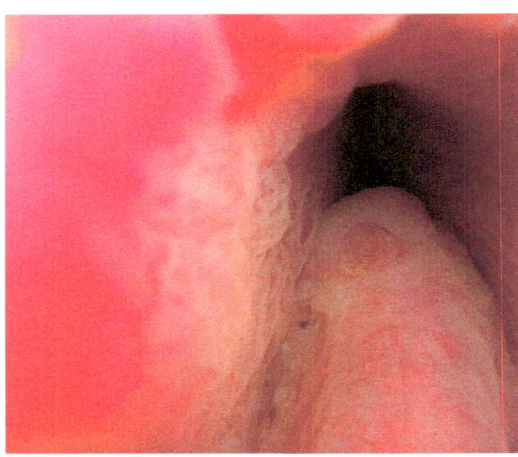

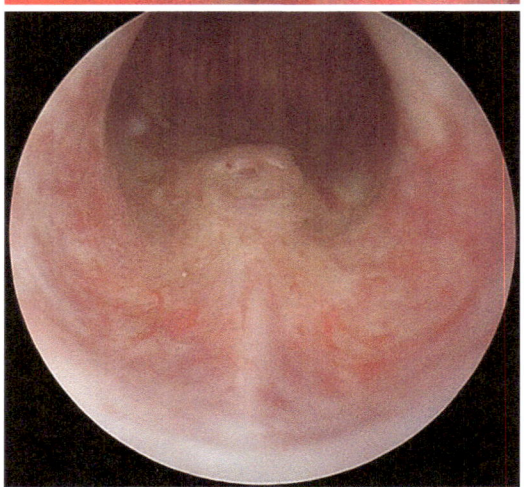

Fig. 2.10 Within the prostatic urethra lumen, the top of the veru is pictured at 6 o'clock with large kissing lateral prostatic urethral lobes superiorly

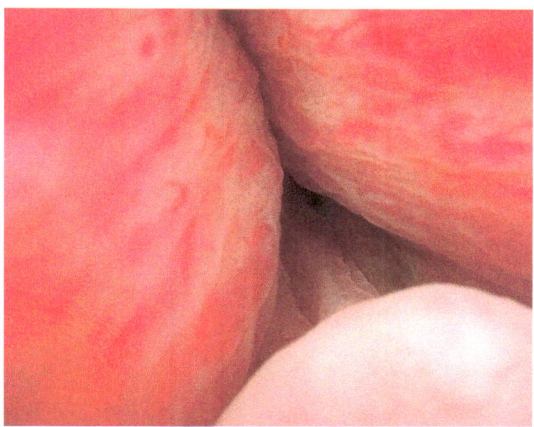

Fig. 2.11 Traversing the large lateral lobes

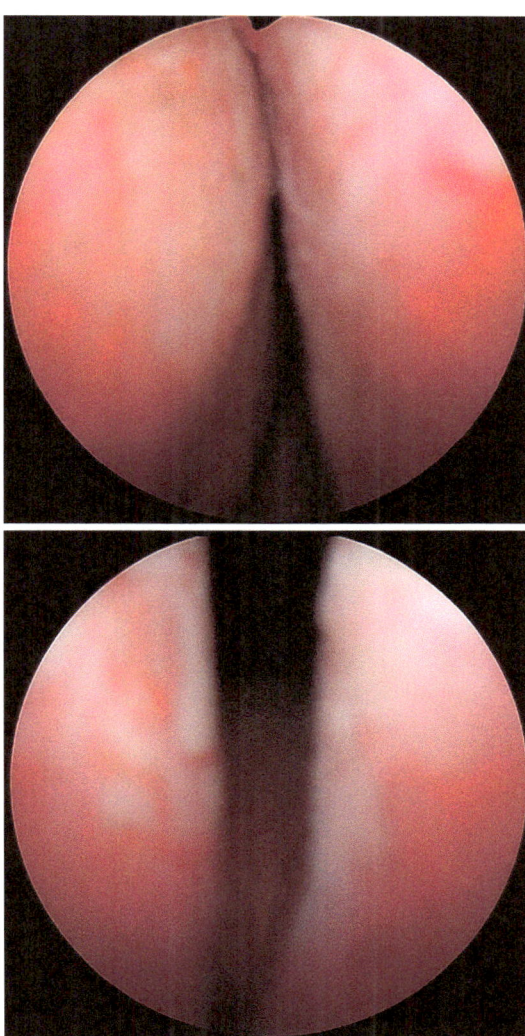

Fig. 2.12 Moderately
large median lobe picture
center extending from the
bladder neck

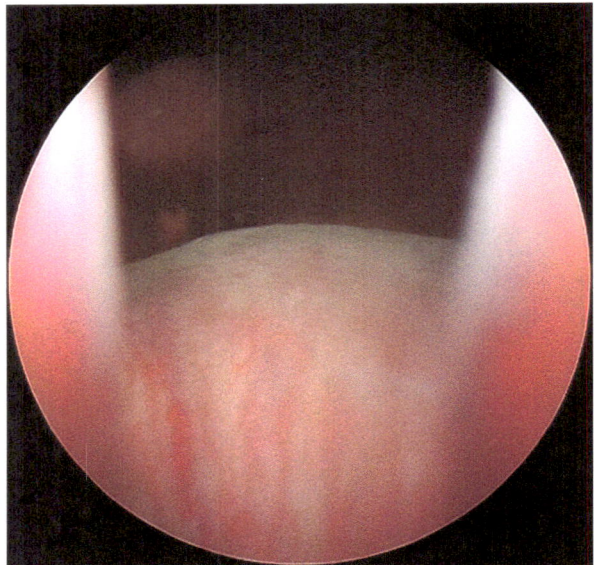

Fig. 2.13 Bladder neck
with no significant
prostatic lobe hypertrophy

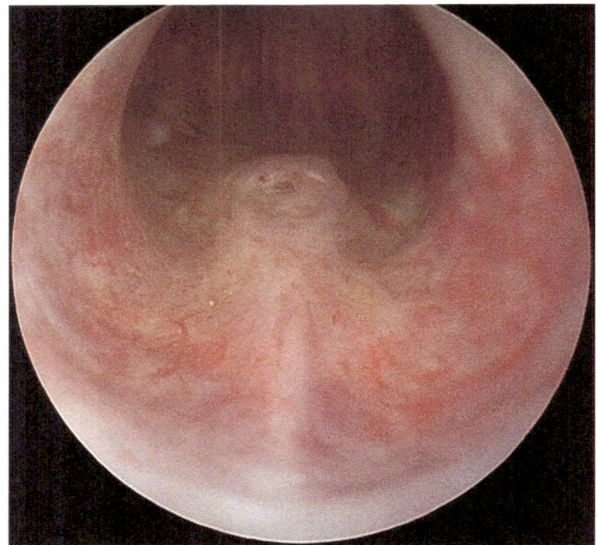

2.2   Female Urethra

2.2.1   Descriptive Anatomy

The female urethra is approximately 4 cm long with an external meatal appearance
of a 5–6 mm anterior orifice. The meatal orifice is located approx. 2 cm inferior to
the clitoris and within the folds of the labia minora. The external urethral meatus has

bordering glands, called Skene glands (periurethral glands), where they are positioned just along the superior lateral aspect [3].

The route of the urethra takes a short forward and downward trajectory from the bladder neck where its midpoint progresses horizontally behind the symphysis pubis. This trajectory has continent implications for the female patient.

Histologically, the urethral mucosa is made up of squamous epithelial cells near the external meatus, pseudo-stratified columnar epithelial cells (predominantly), and transitional epithelial cells along the bladder neck.

Anatomically there is a single sphincter made up of circular striated muscle surrounding the smooth muscle of the urethra, termed the rhabdosphincter. The location of this sphincter is within the proximal two-thirds of the urethra. This sphincter has both a role in voluntary and involuntary continence [4].

2.2.2   Cystoscopic Anatomy

The female urethra is also characterized by two segments, the anterior and posterior portion as it pertains to the dividing sphincteric line, the urogenital diaphragm. Cystoscopically this exact area can be difficult to localize given adequate coaptation throughout and near homogenous appearance of the mucosa. The urethral lumen typically appears as a transverse tract with a longitudinal projection that runs along the entire posterior wall, called the urethral crest [4] (see Figs. 2.14, 2.15, and 2.16).

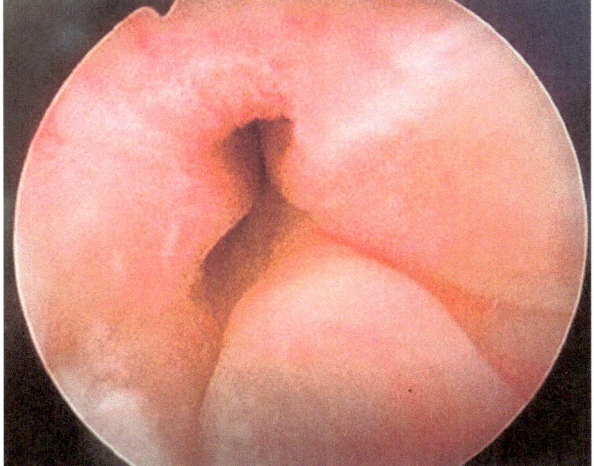

Fig. 2.14 Female urethra after introduction of scope with coaptation of the external sphincter. The urethral crest seen at 6'o clock

Fig. 2.15 Having passed through the sphincter, the bladder neck and the bladder lumen is readily visible

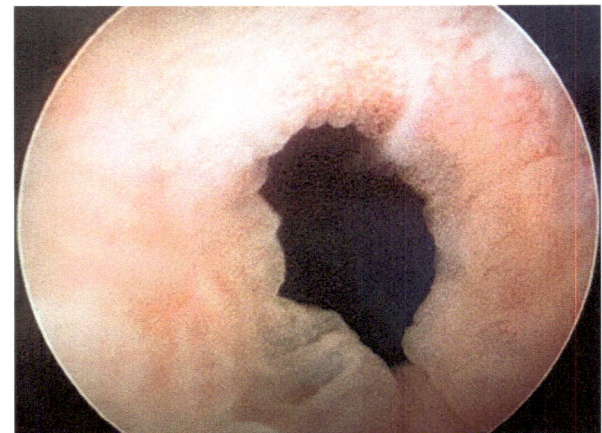

Fig. 2.16 Closer view of the female bladder neck with the bladder lumen beyond

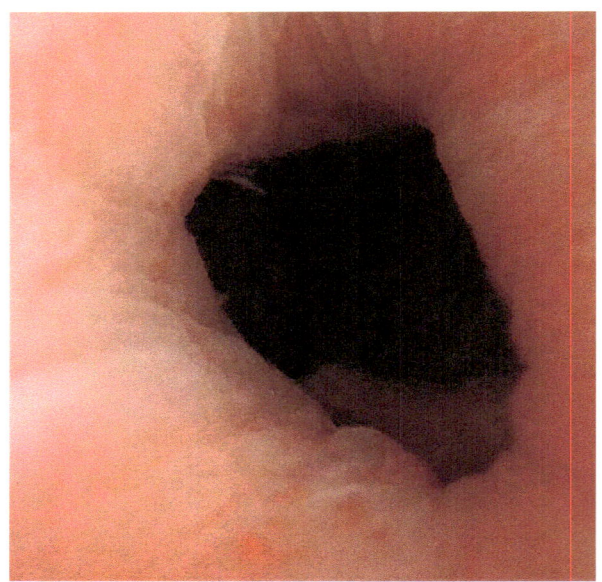

2.3   Bladder

2.3.1   Descriptive Anatomy

Descriptively the bladder is a hollow musculomembranous organ, characterized by four microscopic layers: serous/outer connective tissue, muscle, submucosal connective tissue/lamina propria, and lastly the mucosa/urothelium [5]. The urothelium is a transitional epithelial structure 3–6 cell layers thick. This layer of cells/tissue is what is directly visible on cystoscopic assessment. Beyond the urothelium lies the lamina propria, it is juxtaposed between the basement membrane of the urothelium and the detrusor muscle. The lamina propria is the visceral connective tissue of the organ where the vascular network runs and supplies oxygen to both the muscle and mucosal layers. The bladder's detrusor muscle is composed of three layers: The inner longitudinal, the middle circular, and lastly the outer longitudinal [6].

Anatomically the bladder can be divided into two separate muscular structures, the base versus the body. The bladder base is structurally different because it functions to store urine while the body functions to propel urine upon muscular contraction. This structural difference is exhibited by the differing proportion of muscarinic versus adrenergic receptors within these to muscle zones. The base of the bladder is the thickest portion of the bladder, and it is attached to adjacent structures such as the rectum posteriorly (forming the rectovesical pouch) and the vesical neck and urethra anteriorly. In females, the base is primary in contact with the cervix and anterior vaginal wall (forming the uterovesical pouch). The lateral walls of the bladder are bordered by the obturator internus muscle, along with its fascial layer, bilaterally. Anteriorly the bladder comes into contact with transversalis fascia (endopelvic fascia) that covers the walls and floor of the pelvis. When full, the anterior wall of the bladder comes into direct contact of the posterior surface of the anterior abdominal wall. Lastly, the bladder is suspended by the remains of the urachus; tethered to the umbilicus by the umbilical ligaments. The superior aspect of the bladder borders the peritoneal cavity [3].

2.3.2   Cystoscopic Anatomy

Cystoscopic assessment of the bladder divides the bladder into the following segments: The bladder neck, the superficial trigone, and lastly the bladder walls (see Figs. 2.17, 2.18, 2.19, 2.20, 2.21, and 2.22). Further characterization of the bladder walls will allow for localization of found lesions to either the base/fundus (as the area extending from the inter-ureteric ridge), the lateral walls, the anterior wall, and lastly the dome of the bladder marked by an air bubble that occurred upon introduction of the cystoscope [3].

While using the cystoscope the bladder neck appears as a rounded cylindrical opening, in the absence of prostatic lobe enlargement. The bladder neck opens directly into the bladder's lumen, which should clearly be appreciated with the cystoscope within the prostatic urethra.

The superficial trigone is a triangular structure area on top of the base of the bladder just posterior to the bladder neck extending caudally towards the Veru (see Fig. 2.17). The trigonal ridge can vary in size between a smooth flat raised structure to a more pronounced fold. Along the intraluminal lateral aspects of the trigone are the respective ureteral orifices.

The ureteral orifices appear as an oblique slit or as a patent orifice at the junction of the anterior ureteric ridge and the ureteral bar of the trigone (see Figs. 2.18 and 2.19). During voiding, the superficial trigone draws the orifices distally making the course of the ureter through the vesicle wall more oblique in order to prevent backflow of urine up into the kidneys.

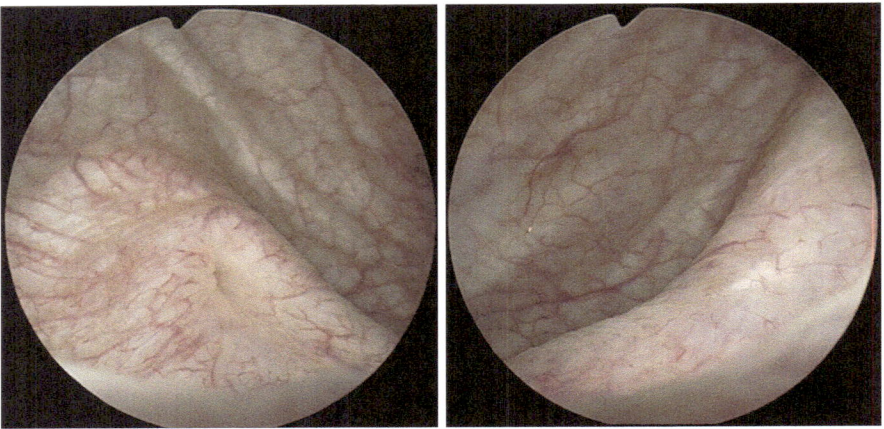

Fig. 2.17 The superficial trigone pictured by two cystoscopic photographs

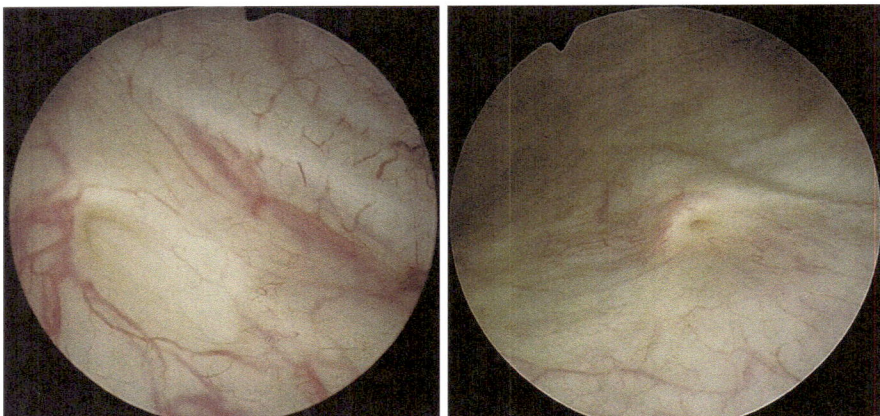

Fig. 2.18 Right ureteral orifices picture above

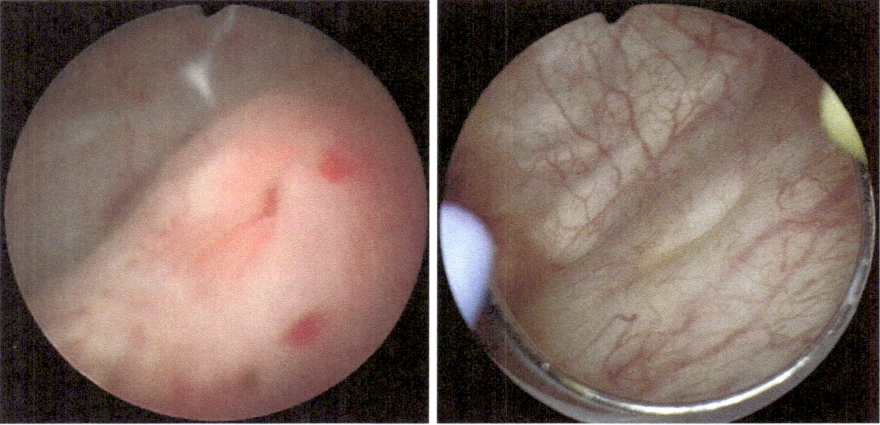

Fig. 2.19 Left ureteral orifices

Fig. 2.20 Lateral walls of the bladder. The right lateral wall (above picture) and the left later wall (below picture)

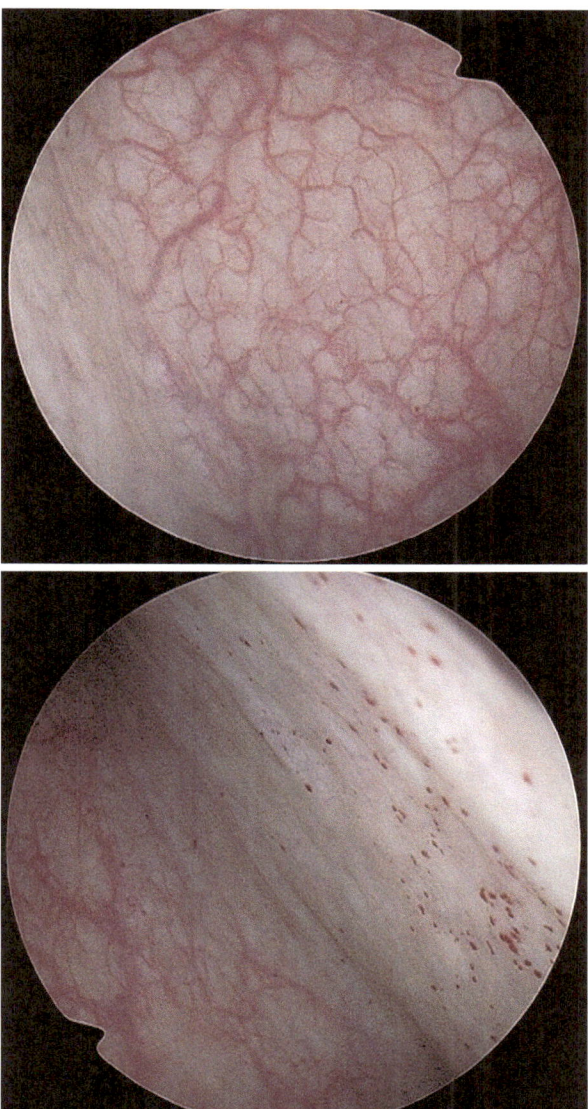

Fig. 2.21 Posterior wall

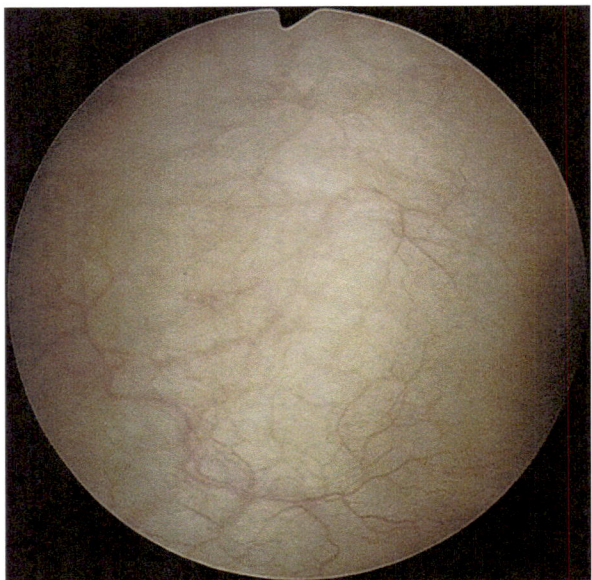

Fig. 2.22 Dome of the
bladder is marked by the
location of the air bubble
following introduction of
the cystoscope

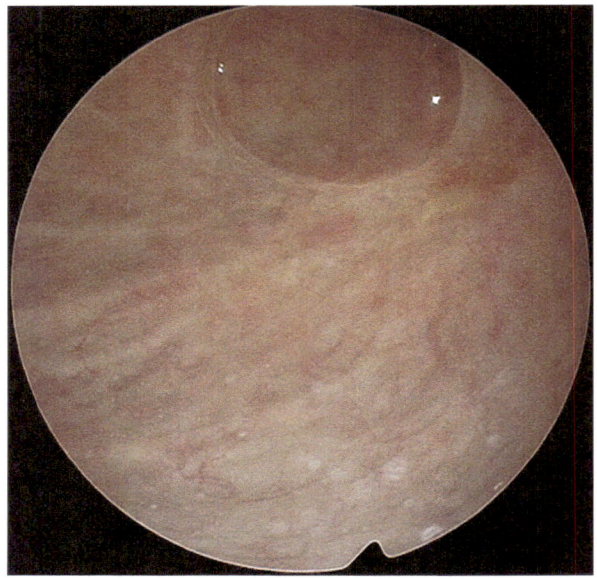

The bladder's wall or shape will appear different depending upon the level of distention of the bladder. When the bladder is partially filled or empty, the view from the cystoscope will have numerous mucosal folds versus the flat mucosal appearance with near complete distention (see Figs. 2.23 and 2.24). The appearance of the superficial layer of the bladder, the mucosa, is usually translucent yellow or pale pink allowing for direct visualization of the submucosal vascular network.

Fig. 2.23 The bladder
when not fully distended,
as evidenced by rugae and
incomplete distention

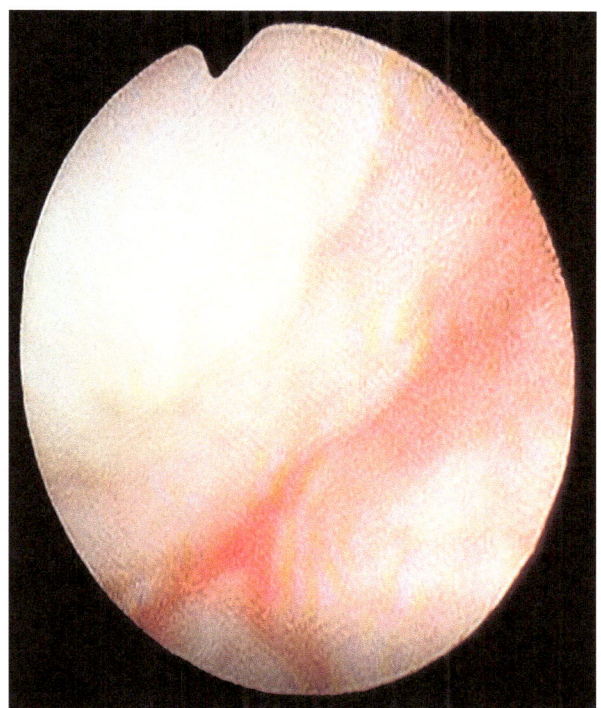

Fig. 2.24 Nearly a
complete evacuated
bladder

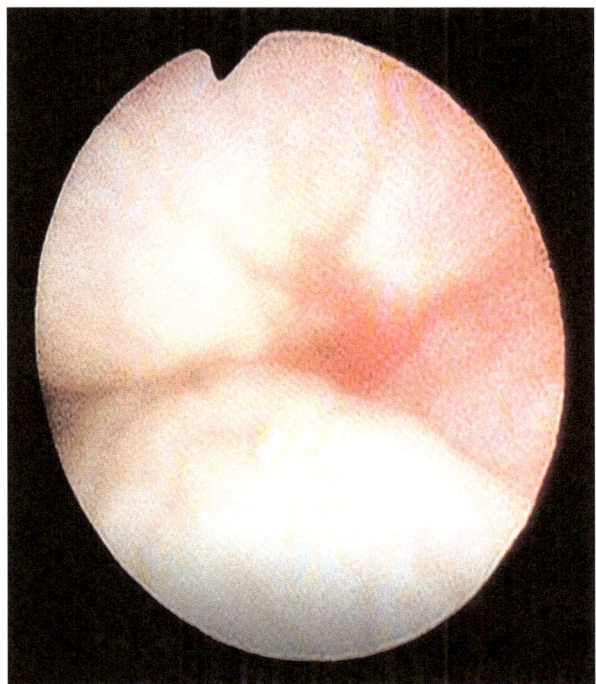

2.4   Normal Anatomical Variants

This section will briefly detail normal variations in the urethra and bladder. In order to distinctly separate this section from benign pathology, this section will only pertain to congenital anatomical variants.

2.4.1   Common Urethral Anatomical Variants

2.4.1.1   Hypospadias

It is characterized by the failure of the urethra to fully mature in fetal development so that its site of termination is on the anterior aspect of the glans penis. The urethral meatus in a hypospadias patient is located along the ventral line anywhere proximally to where it is found in complete differentiation.

2.4.1.2   Epispadias/Exstrophy

Analogous to the hypospadias, this condition is also secondary to incomplete differentiation. With epispadias, the urethral meatus occurs along the dorsal aspect of the penis. Exstrophy, is a more severe termination of maturation with varying degrees of bladder, intestinal, and urethral involvement.

2.4.1.3   Urethral Valve

Posterior urethral valves are classified either as type 1, 2, or 3 depending upon the valve structure and the relation to the veru in the male infant. The hypothesis for formation is thought to be due to failure of regression of the terminal segment of the mesonephric duct [7].This condition is typically diagnosed prior to birth or early in a patient's life/childhood.

2.4.1.4   Enlarged Prostatic Utricle

The prostatic utricle is a congenital 1 cm indention in the prostatic urethra on the veru. This indention is actually the homologue of the uterus and vagina, derived from the paramesonephric duct [7]. When enlarged, the prostatic utricle may accommodate the advancement of the cystoscope by at least 2 cm. It is commonly associated with a hypospadias.

2.4.2   Common Bladder Anatomical Variants

2.4.2.1   Ureteral Duplication with/without Ectopic Orifice

Ureteral duplication on diagnostic cystoscopy will be appreciated as an additional ureteral orifice. Other forms of ureteral duplication, such as a bifid or incomplete duplication, would only be appreciable on retrograde pyelogram or ureteroscopy.

An ectopic ureter by definition, will not enter the bladder along the trigone, with the likely occurrence of an orifice contained within the posterior urethra. In a duplicated system, this commonly involves the upper pole. This is secondary to a later budding/development of the upper renal moiety in comparison to the lower pole. In females, the ectopic ureter can have its orifice along the vestibule, the anterior vaginal wall, and the uterus or cervix. Both males and females can have an ectopic ureter enter within the rectum. These later organ structures would not be surveyed on diagnostic cystoscopy, but rather the problem would be caught on radiographic urography [8].

2.4.3   Ureterocele

A ureterocele is a cystic dilation of the distal/terminal ureter, adjacent to the ureteral orifice, that in its "simple" form causes a protrusion of the ureter into the bladder without any upper tract dilatation (see Fig. 2.25). This will typically appear as a bulge on the ureteral orifice. Ureteroceles are however known to be associated with hydronephrosis secondary to obstruction.

Fig. 2.25 Left ureterocele with small crowning ureteral stone

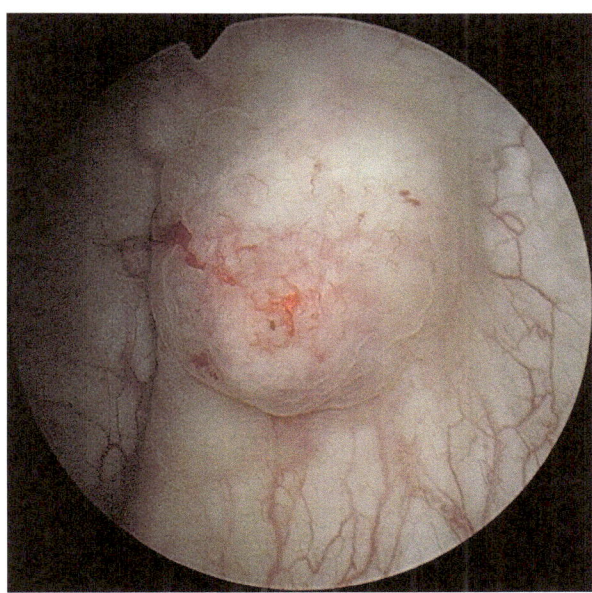

Ectopic ureteroceles do occur, although less common, and are characterized by some portion of the ureterocele traveling through the bladder neck or urethra (the cystic tract undermines into these areas) (see Fig. 2.26). In these instances, the ureteral orifice can also remain in the bladder.

Photobank of normal anatomy: Internal lower urinary tract anatomy (Figs. 2.27, 2.28, 2.29, 2.30, 2.31, 2.32, 2.33, 2.34, 2.35, and 2.36).

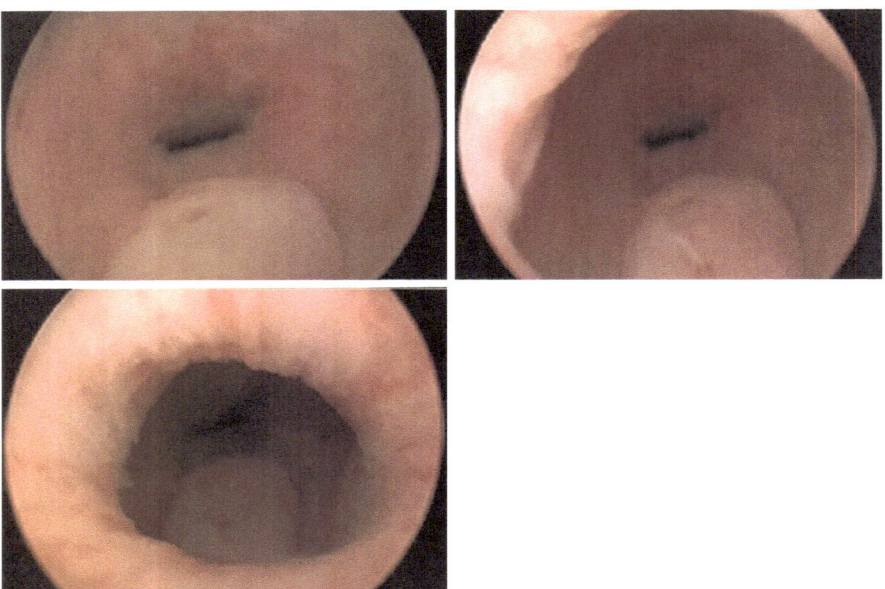

Fig. 2.26 Pictured above is an ectopic ureterocele within the mid portion of female urethra. The photo was provided by the Urogynecology team at Atrium health

Fig. 2.27 The male bulbar urethra, where the urethra begins to curve anterior towards the external sphincter and the prostatic urethra

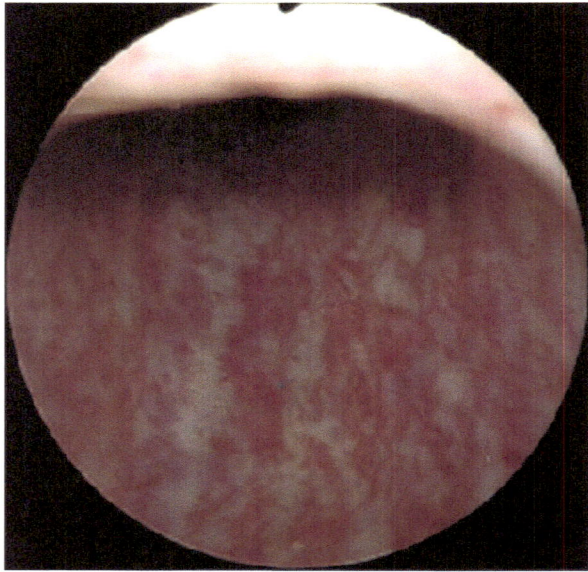

Fig. 2.28 Hyperemic male external sphincter. The clinician had to flex the scope superiorly in order to directly visualize the center of the sphincter/lumen

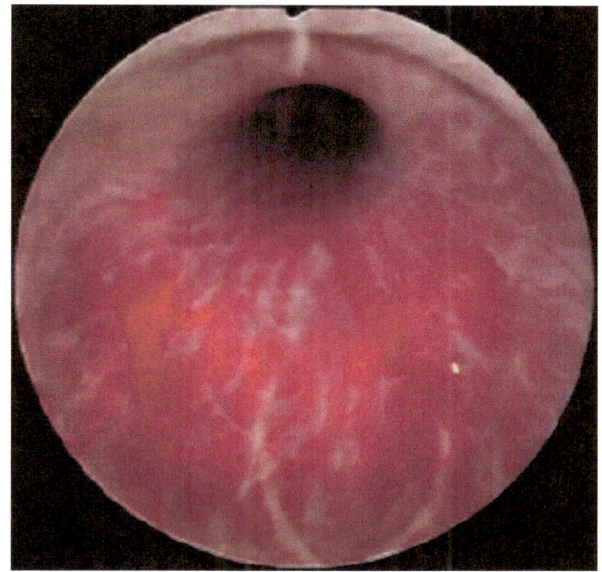

Fig. 2.29 Right ureter seen with a distal curl of a double "J" ureteral stent

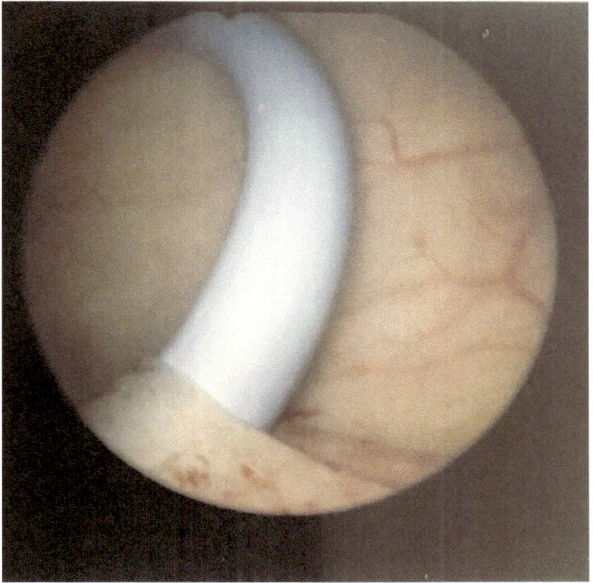

Fig. 2.30 Pendoulous urethra, with evidence of urethritis secondary to instrumentation. The two black lines seen here are from a double "J" ureteral stent suture that allows for self removal

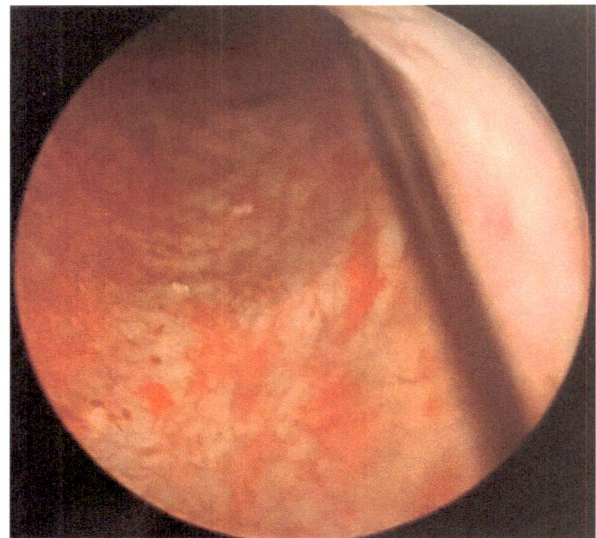

Fig. 2.31 Male bulbar urethra with a dangler double "J" suture seen exiting the external sphincter

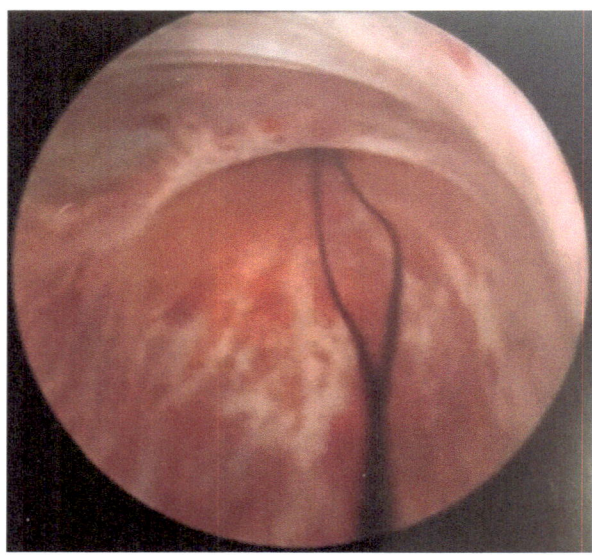

Fig. 2.32 Double "J" dangler suture seen exiting the external urinary sphincter of a male patient

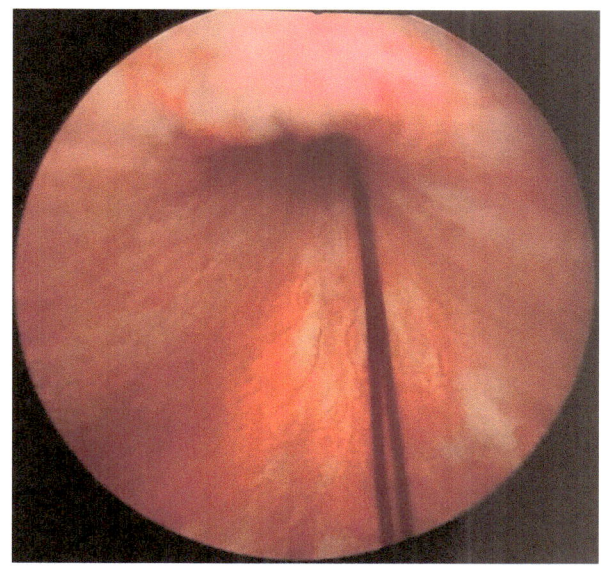

Fig. 2.33 Enlarged bilateral lateral lobes of the prostatic urethra. Seen posterior to the lobes is the median lob and bladder neck

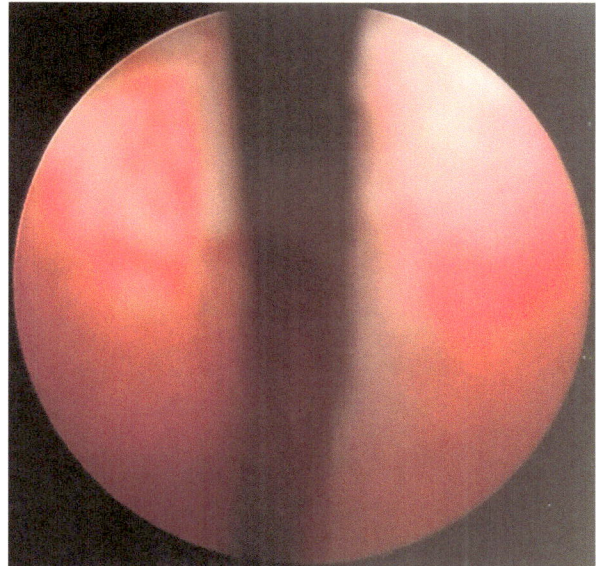

Fig. 2.34 The bladder neck and lumen coming into visualization. The base of the bladder is noted to be obscured by a prominent median lobe and high bladder neck

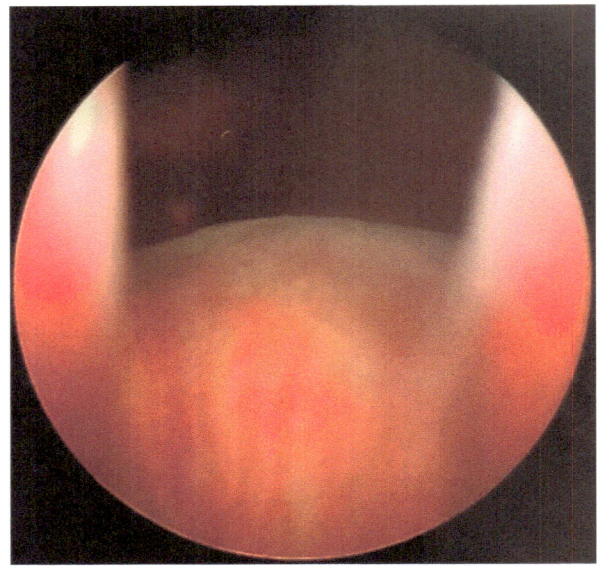

Fig. 2.35 Obstructing lateral lobes of a prostatic urethra. This patient had significant obstructive lower urinary tract symptoms

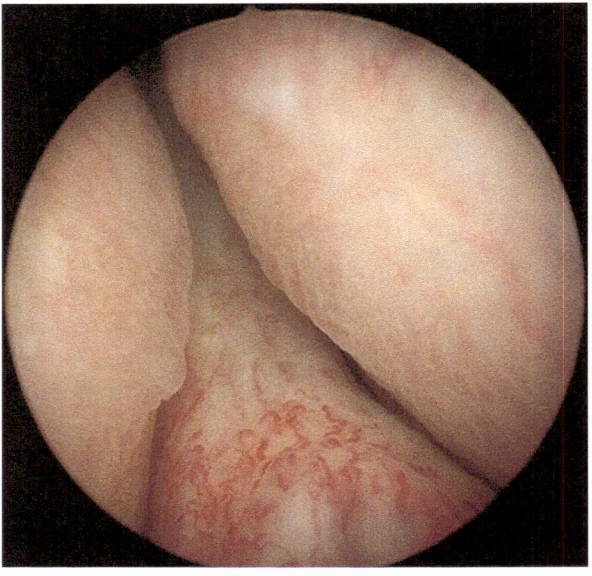

Fig. 2.36 Retroflexion
assessment of the bladder
neck. Noted enlarged
protruding median lobe
extending into the bladder.
Photo provided by Dr.
Mark Makhuli at Atrium
Health

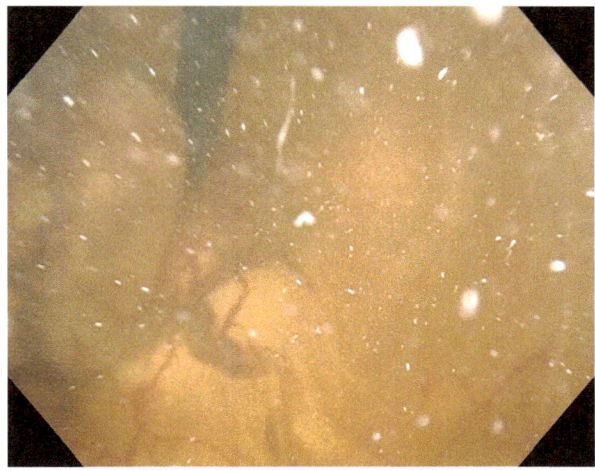

References

1. Moore R, Bishoff PJ, Loening S, Docimo S. Minimally invasive urologic surgery. New York: Taylor & Francis; 2005.
2. Nita G, Geavlete P. Endoscopic aspects of prostate. In: Geavlete P, editor. Endoscopic diagnosis and treatment in prostate pathology. Oxford: Elsevier Incorporated; 2016.
3. MacLennan G. Female genital tract and urethra. In: MacLennan G, editor. Hinman's Atlast of UroSurgical anatomy. Philadelphia: Saunders; 2012. p. 287–304.
4. Multescu R, Alexandrescu E, Geavlete. Anatomy of the urethra. In: Geavlete P, editor. Endoscopic diagnosis and treatment in urethral pathology. Oxford: Elsevier; 2016.
5. Crafts RC. Abdominopelvic cavity and perineum. A Textbook of Human Anatomy. Hoboken, NJ: John Wiley & Sons Inc; 1985. p. 335–58.
6. MacLennan G. Bladder, ureterovesical junction, and rectum. In: MacLennan G, editor. Hinman's atlas of UroSurgical anatomy. Philadelphia: Saunders; 2012. p. 211–48.
7. Casale P, Canning D. Congenital anomalies. In: Hanno P, Guzzo T, Malkowicz B, Wein A, editors. Penn clinical manual of urology. Philadelphia: Saunders; 2014. p. 840–83.
8. MacLennan G. Kidney, ureter, and adrenal glands. In: MacLennan G, editor. Hinman's atlas of UroSurgical anatomy. Philadelphia: Saunders; 2012. p. 151–210.

Chapter 3
Benign Urethral Pathology

3.1 Urethritis

3.1.1 Pathophysiology

Urethritis by definition is the inflammation of the urethra. This is a common ailment experienced by both men and women. In fact, urinary tract infections are listed as one of the leading causes for patients to visit their primary care provider. The inflammation is usually secondary to infection by a bacterial organism; however, other eukaryotic microorganisms and viruses have been implicated. Lastly, inflammation can also occur secondary to genitourinary irritants.

Infections occur due to a failure or breakdown in host defense mechanisms when additionally exposed to a virulent organism. Host defense mechanisms include the normal inhibitory and bactericidal effects of urine (pH, enzymes, etc.), normal voiding, and adequate estrogen levels for vaginal mucosa. Lastly, bacteria have evolved over time in order to overcome these preventative measures, such as by increasing the variety of cell surface adhesion molecules and changing the microscopic environment (Proteus species, Klebsiella species, and *Staphylococcus saprophyticus* produce urease, causing an increase in urine pH) [1].

Inflammation caused by nonbacterial organisms is unlikely to appear different upon macroscopic/cystoscopic assessment. Inflammation is a generalized immune response, and thus the presence of inflammatory polyps, erythema, and/or swelling should suggest that an infection may be present. Bacterial infections, however, are the most common cause of urethral infection, although the herpes simplex virus has been implicated in causing urethritis. STIs, such as *Chlamydia trachomatis*, and *Neisseria gonorrhoeae* are known to cause isolated urethritis.

© The Author(s), under exclusive license to Springer Nature
Switzerland AG 2022
B. C. Tenny, M. O'Neill, *Diagnostic Cystoscopy*,
https://doi.org/10.1007/978-3-031-10668-2_3

3.1.2 Clinical Presentation

Symptoms suggestive of urethritis include burning with/without urination. Urethritis typically co-occurs with cystitis, and thus there are additional complaints of urinary frequency, painful urination, and possible gross hematuria. If a patient reports vaginal itching, dyspareunia, and/or vaginal discharge, the clinician should have a higher suspicion of vaginitis. Urethral discharge is commonly present in STIs; gonorrhea and chlamydia can cause a clear to white discharge.

Laboratory workup will typically reveal some combination of the following: pyuria, bacteriuria, dipstick + nitrites, and dipstick + leukocyte esterase. It is important to obtain an adequate clean catch specimen and possibly a catheterized one if there is any doubt on which anatomical structure is inflamed. If urine culture fails to identify a culprit organism, the clinician should consider testing for sexually transmitted diseases in sexually active patients.

Sexually transmitted infections are one of the most common reported infectious diseases in the US. Organisms can typically be diagnosed by immediate gram stain from a urethral swab/smear. Under microscope, Gonorrhea will appear as intracellular gram-negative diplococci in polymorphonuclear leukocytes, and chlamydia also an intracellular gram-negative bacterium but usually bacilli shaped. Alternative available testing for STIs include nucleic acid molecular amplification tests (NAATs), polymerase chain reaction (PCR), and strand displacement amplification (SDA), all of which measure DNA and/or RNA. These tests thus can remain positive for an organism, even approx. 3 weeks post eradication, due to residual DNA. The clinician should thus consider waiting at least a month prior to testing for a cure [2].

Although STIs are a known cause of isolated urethritis, not involving bladder infection, they are complicated by approx. 50% of gonorrhea and chlamydia being asymptomatic [2]. Therefore, the CDC recommends annual screening for all women under the age of 25, all pregnant women, and older women with multiple sex partners.

3.1.3 Cystoscopic Image(s)

3.1.4 Suggested Treatments

Empirical treatment for a urinary tract infection is appropriate and does not necessarily warrant a urine culture for diagnosis. Duration of antimicrobial therapy is tailored towards the suspected organism and the chosen antibiotic.

Antibiotics:

Nitrofurantoin 100 mg PO BID for 5 days.

Trimethoprim-sulfamethoxazole 800 mg/160 mg PO BID for 3–5 days.

Cephalexin/cephalosporins 250 mg PO QID for 3 to 5 days.

Ciprofloxacin/fluoroquinolones 500 mg PO BID for 3 days.

Fosfomycin, single 3gm IM single dose.

Treatment for Sexually Transmitted Infections:

Gonorrhea

Ceftriaxone 250 mg IM single dose.

Cefixime 400 mg PO single dose.

Azithromycin 2gm PO single dose (pregnant).

*It is recommended that the treatment for coinfection with chlamydia be implemented given the cost of subsequent testing and the risk of complication of pelvic inflammatory disease if left untreated.

Chlamydia

Azithromycin 1gm PO single dose.

Doxycycline 100 mg PO BID for 7 days.

Erythromycin 500 mg PO QID for 7 days.

Summary Key Points

- Bacterial infections, the most common cause of urethral infection. Additionally consider STIs for isolated urethritis.
- Cardinal symptom of burning with/without urination.
- Labs: UA, urine culture, gram stain, NAATs/PCR/SDA for STIs (can remain positive 3 weeks post eradication).

  - All women under the age of 25, all pregnant women, and older women with multiple sex partners should have annual screening for gonorrhea and chlamydia (CDC recommendation).

- *Cystoscopic appearance:* Turbid or purulent urine, erythema to mucosa, possible edematous polyps, and some sloughing of mucosal lining (see Fig. 3.1, 3.2, and 3.3).
- Tx with empiric antibiotics.

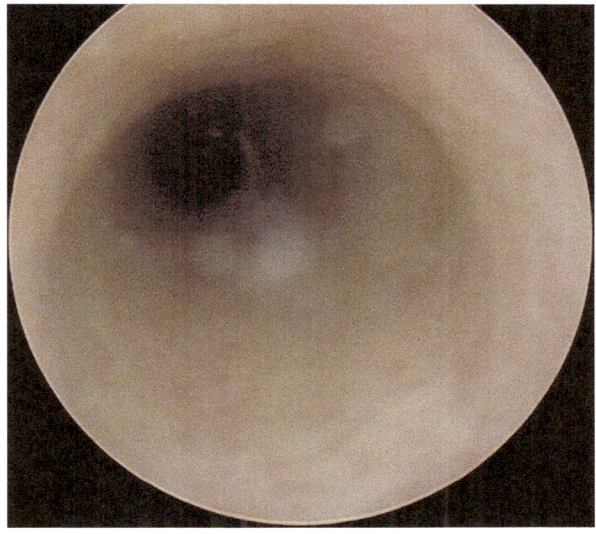

Fig. 3.1 Male pendulous urethra with turbid/cloudy urine

Fig. 3.2 Closer
examination of the mucosa
demonstrates inflammatory
changes of the urethra

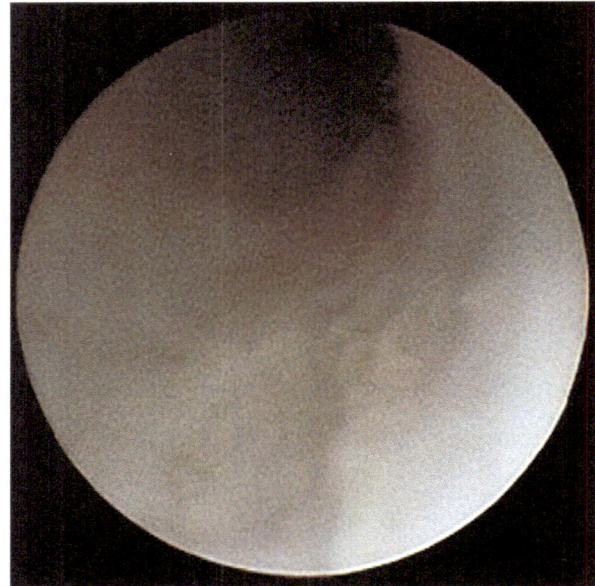

Fig. 3.3 Male pendulous
urethra with evident
erythema of the mucosa

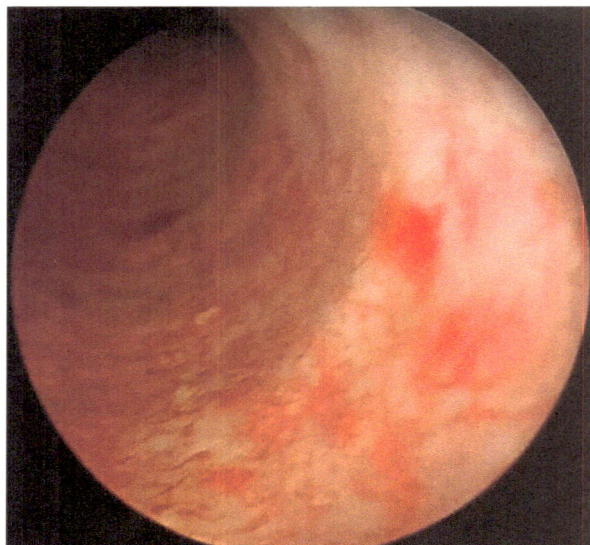

Additional References for Consideration

- Penn Clinical Manual of Urology by Philip M. Hanno MD, MPH, Thomas J. Guzzo MD, MPH, S. Bruce Malkowicz MD and Alan J. Wein MD, FACS, PhD.
- Textbook of Family Medicine by Robert E. Rakel MD and David P. Rakel MD.

3.2 Urethral Stricture Disease

3.2.1 Pathophysiology

An acquired urethral stricture, or plainly termed urethral scar tissue, develops secondary to acute or chronic inflammation resulting in a narrower caliber and inelasticity of the urethral lumen. Urethral strictures can also be congenital and are due to abnormal fusion between the anterior and posterior urethra. Inflammation that causes acquired stricture disease occurs from either trauma, infection, or ischemic injury.

Urethral stricture disease has a male preponderance rarely occurring in females. This has likely resulted in the limited number of available studies able to accurately quantify the incidence of female urinary obstruction. For example, a study by Blavias and Groutz assessed video urodynamics in 587 females and only 38 met their diagnostic criteria for outlet obstruction. Of those who met this criterion only 13% had urethral stricture disease. The predominant cause of urinary obstruction in females was found to be secondary to severe pelvic organ prolapse and prior anti-incontinence surgery [3].

3.2.2 Clinical Presentation

Patients will present with report of obstructive lower urinary tract symptoms. This can include any combination of the following: urinary frequency, slow urinary stream, straining to void, incomplete bladder emptying, painful urination, hematuria, flank pain, and incontinence. Stenosis/stricture disease of the urethral meatus can cause splitting of urinary stream.

Diagnostic workup can include radiography, cystourethroscopy, and in-office functional voiding studies (see Fig. 3.4). Identification of meatal stenosis can be made by assessment of the external genitalia. In-office functional tests may include post-void residual and urine flowmetry. Anterior urethral strictures may require retrograde urethrogram (RUG) and/or voiding cystourethrogram (VCUG) for identification (see Fig. 3.5). Both modalities used together can assist with characterizing the length of the scar tissue for operative planning. Cystourethroscopy allows for direct visualization of the most distal aspect of the scar and can possibly assist in setting up for treatment.

Fig. 3.4 Urologist
interpretation of the above
retrograde urethrogram:
This shows a focal stricture
disease extending over
much of the proximal
pendulous and majority of
the bulbar urethra. Note the
small caliber of the urethra
throughout

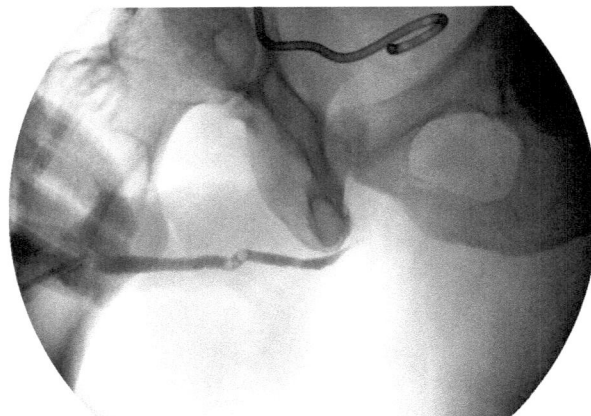

Fig. 3.5 Urologist
interpretation of a
retrograde urethrogram:
RUG is demonstrating a
narrow caliber mid- to
proximal bulbar stricture,
about a centimeter in
length

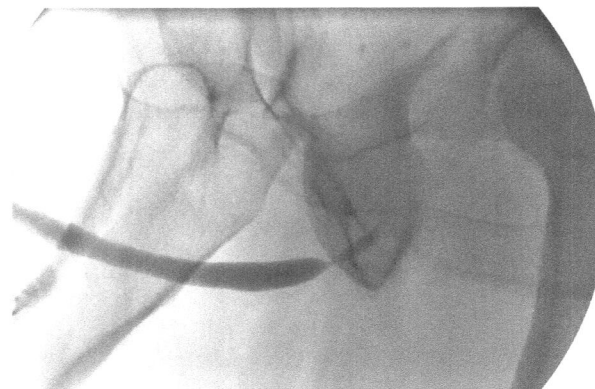

3.2.2.1 Cystoscopic Images

3.2.3 Suggested Treatments

The treatment of urethral stricture disease is changing as new literature demonstrates the possible benefit of delayed reconstruction over immediate dilation. Immediate dilation certainly treats the acute obstruction; however, long-term studies have demonstrated a durable success rate of only approx. 30–50% [4].

3.2.3.1 Immediate Dilation

Performed upon immediate identification of stricture disease. Preferably performed with some local anesthetic infused lubrication. Tools for dilation are numerous, including but not limited to, urethral sounds, filiform and followers, and sequential over the wire urethral dilators. There is risk of injury, given the blind but assisted passage of dilator, that may result in a more complex scar.

3.2.3.2 Direct Vision Incisional Urethrotomy (DVIU)

DVIU is a procedure performed under general anesthesia while using a rigid cysto-scope. A cold knife incises the scar at 12 o'clock, and a catheter is typically left in place for 3–10 days post procedure for reepithelization. Short-term, <6 months, suc-cess fates are robust; however, as previously mentioned, long-term success rates are less than 30% [5]. Attempts to prolong a dilated urethral caliber have been made with scheduled self-catheterizing by patients under clinician recommendation. This procedure should only be performed on scar tissues that are less than 2 cm.

3.2.3.3 Reconstructive Surgery/Urethroplasty

Involves excision of the scared urethra with either end to end anastomosis or buccal substation. End to end anastomosis is a viable option in stricture disease measuring less than 2 cm. Long-term success rates have been reported at 85–90%.

Summary Key Points
- Common etiology of acquired urethral stricture disease: infection, trauma, or ischemia.
- Present with obstructive lower urinary tract symptoms.
- Diagnostics: RUG for anterior urethral strictures. VCUG for proximal urethral strictures. PVR and Uroflometry may additionally be helpful.
- *Cystoscopic appearance:* Evident narrowing of urethral lumen with/without impediment to traversing with the cystoscope. May be solitary or multiple, and large caliber or completely obliterative (see Figs. 3.6, 3.7, 3.8, 3.9, and 3.10).
- Treatment: Immediate dilation versus delayed reconstruction with SPT.

Fig. 3.6 Concentric stricture seen in the pendulous urethra

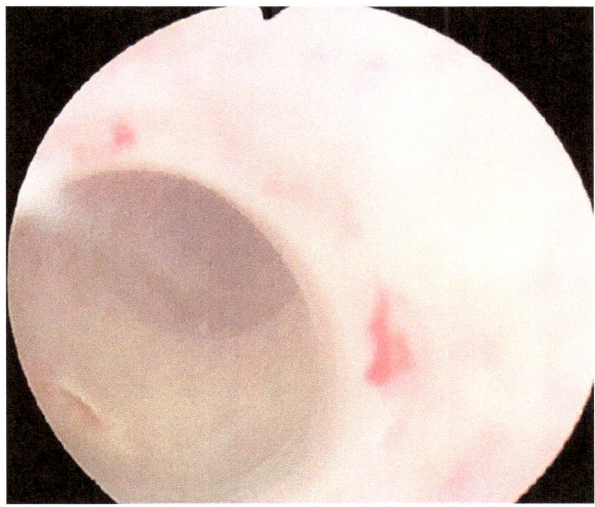

Fig. 3.7 Concentric thin
stricture. Large caliber
accommodating the 16fr
flexible cystoscope

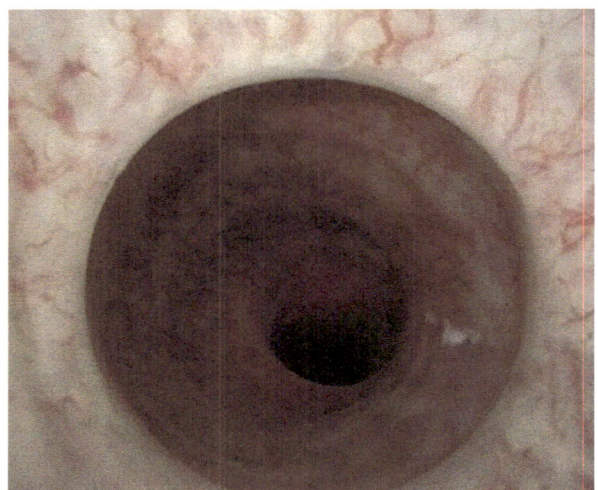

Fig. 3.8 Tight concentric
urethral stricture with
sensor guide wire
accessing the bladder

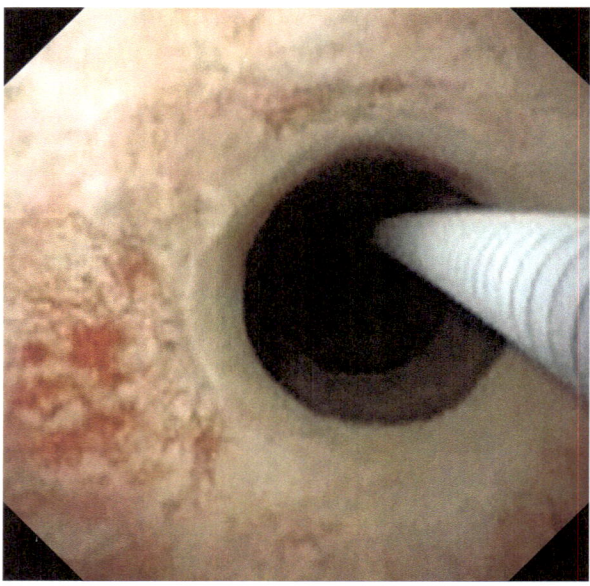

Fig. 3.9 Pinpoint membranous urethral stricture

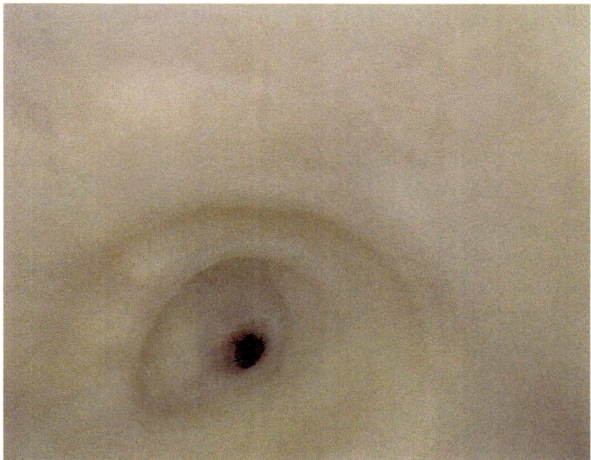

Fig. 3.10 Complete obliteration of the urethral lumen at the membranous urethra

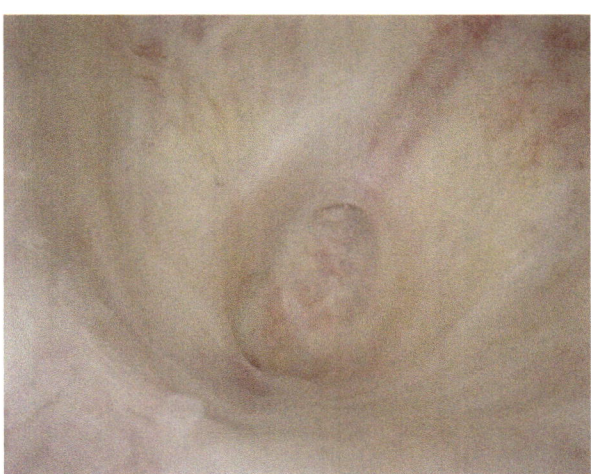

- Immediate dilation- durable success of approx. 30–50%.

    Will likely require DVIU (<30% long term success after 6 months).
    Best if stricture disease <2 cm.

- Delayed reconstruction with SPT/Urethroplasty- long term success 85–90%.

Additional Books for Consideration
- Penn Clinical Manual of Urology by Philip M. Hanno MD, MPH, Thomas J. Guzzo MD, MPH, S. Bruce Malkowicz MD and Alan J. Wein MD, FACS, PhD.
- Campbell-Walsh-Wein Urology by Alan W. Partin MD, PhD, Roger R. Dmochowski D, MMHC, FACS, Louis R. Kavoussi MD, MBA, and Craig A. Peters M.

3.3   Bladder Neck Contracture

3.3.1   Pathophysiology

Bladder Neck Contracture is a posterior urethral stricture disease process that occurs as an adverse effect of prostatic surgery. The constricting stricture can occur after transurethral resection of the prostate, but most predominantly occurs with prostatectomy (3% versus approx. 5–10% respectively) [4]. This incidence is reported to be decreasing as operative procedures become standardized. Intraoperative and postoperative complications that increase the likelihood of contracture are inadequate approximation of the anastomosis, urine extravasation, and formation of hematoma at the anastomosis.

3.3.2   Clinical Presentation

Symptomatology from a bladder neck contracture is virtually the same as urethral stricture disease, albeit there is a documented or reported history of prostate surgery. Patients will have obstructive lower urinary tract symptoms.

Workup and imaging additionally consists of similar studies. A post void residual and urine flowmetry would document the degree of obstruction in the office. Cystoscopy would identify the constricting scar proximal to the membranous urethra, prior to entrance into the bladder. A VCUG could also help characterize the contracture, however a retrograde urethrogram would be insufficient. On rest the external sphincter, that sits distal to the prostate, is closed preventing retrograde injected contrast from reaching this location.

3.3.3   Cystoscopic Image(s)

3.3.4   Suggested Treatments

Treatment of a bladder neck contracture are reminiscent of other urethral stricture interventions. DVIU can be performed, usually more involved with incising at 3, 6, 9, and 12 o'clock followed by catheterization, although as with urethral stricture disease long term success rates are not the majority. Reconstructive surgery can either be open or robotic (becoming more prevalent) with an abdominoperineal approach given the proximal proximity of the bladder neck. Open perineal incisions are insufficient at reaching this anatomical area. Incontinence is a known complication of repair and sometimes requires the insertion of an artificial urinary sphincter.

Summary Key Points
- Occurs following surgery on the prostate.
- Present with obstructive lower urinary tract symptoms.
- Diagnostics: Cystoscopy gold standard. Uroflometry and PVR can aid in narrowing differential.
- Cystoscopic appearance: Constricting scar proximal to the membranous urethra, prior to entrance into the bladder. If patient had prostatectomy versus large TURP, there will be no prostatic urethra (see Figs. 3.11, 3.12, and 3.13).
- Treatment: Options range from cystoscopic incision of the scar tissue to reconstructive surgery. Surgery will likely require abdominoperineal approach. Open perineal incision is insufficient. The known complication of treatment is stress incontinence.

Additional Books for Consideration
- Penn Clinical Manual of Urology by Philip M. Hanno MD, MPH, Thomas J. Guzzo MD, MPH, S. Bruce Malkowicz MD, and Alan J. Wein MD, FACS, PhD.
- Campbell-Walsh-Wein Urology by Alan W. Partin MD, PhD, Roger R. Dmochowski D, MMHC, FACS, Louis R. Kavoussi MD, MBA, and Craig A. Peters M.

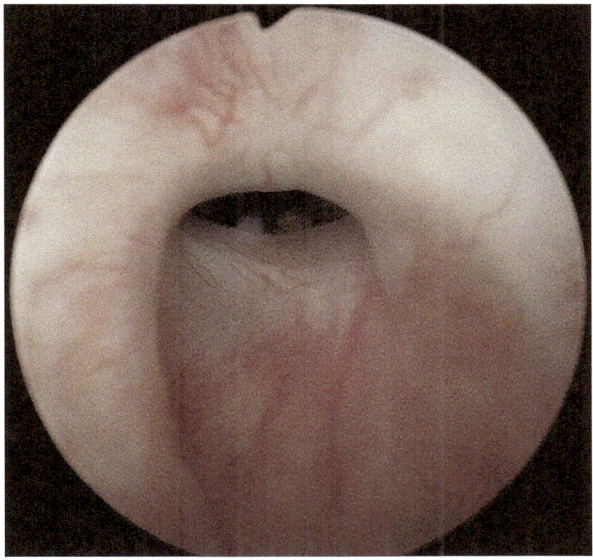

Fig. 3.11 Patient presented with complaints of diminished flow in the setting of TURP history for BPH. Cystoscopy confirmed suspicion of a bladder neck contracture

Fig. 3.12 Bladder neck contracture. Erythema and bleeding seen is secondary to mild urethral dilation in order to get the cystoscope into the bladder

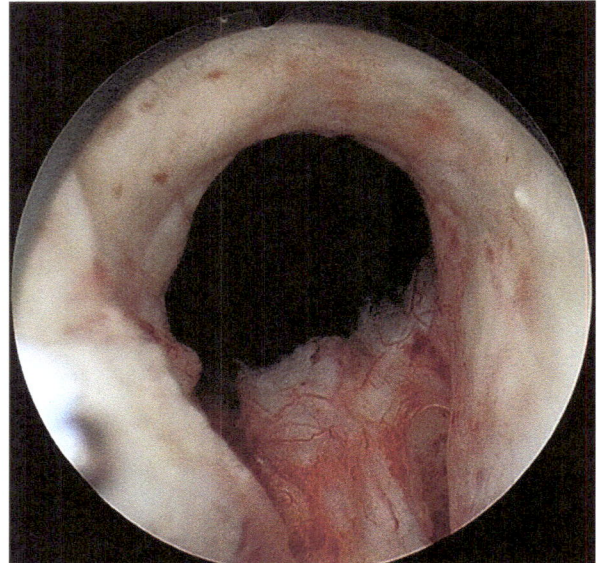

Fig. 3.13 Bladder neck contracture with resultant bladder stone formation

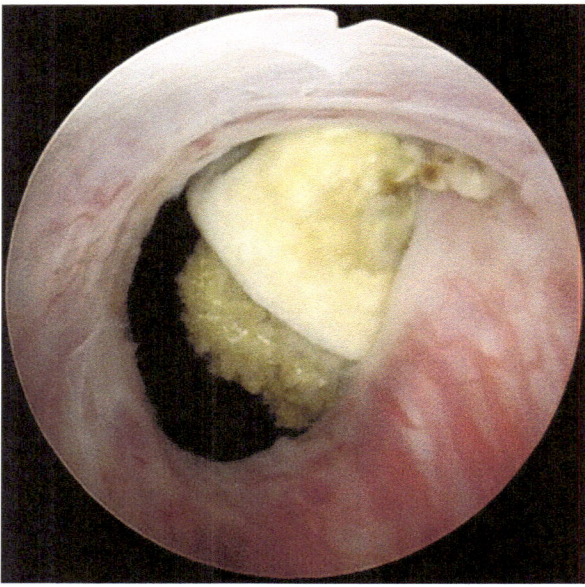

3.4   Benign Prostatic Hyperplasia

3.4.1   Pathophysiology

Benign prostatic hyperplasia (BPH) is a result of cumulative exposure due to circulating androgens produced by the adult male. Normal prostate size/volume has been measured to be approximately 25 ml at age 30 and 35-40 ml at age 80 [6]. An enlarged prostate can vary in size exceeding volumes greater than 100 cc. Interestingly, the size of the prostate does not linearly correlate with severity of symptoms or urodynamic evidence of bladder outlet obstruction. This is primarily due to the peripheral zone making up nearly 75% of total glandular volume. In essence, if the gland grows outward, it would unlikely impact the lumen of the urethra. The central zone makes up the remaining 25% of the functioning glandular prostate and covers the urethra, which is then covered by the peripheral zone laterally and the fibromuscular stroma anteriorly. The functioning glandular portion of the prostate is where the hyperplasia and growth occur; this hyperplastic growth tends to be in a nodular fashion. Nodules form within the central zone causing obstruction as they protrude inward through the smooth muscle and mucosal layers of the proximal urethra.

3.4.2   Clinical Presentation

Patients with benign prostatic hyperplasia may or may not report lower urinary tract symptoms. Those that are experiencing symptoms typically report decrease in urinary stream, hesitancy, straining to void, and terminal dribbling. These symptoms are voiding/emptying symptoms and were previously categorized as obstructive symptoms.

Simple urodynamic testing can be done performed in the clinic with uroflometry and residual urine volumes. Uroflometry uses flow rate to indicate whether there is an impediment to outflow, a prostate obstruction, and is diagnosed if peak flow rate is less than 15 ml/s. 10–15 ml/s is an inconclusive result and consideration for symptomatology should weigh on the decision to treat. Importantly, the recorded curve of the outflow should help in determining whether the test was sufficiently performed. Outlet obstruction is best characterized as "poor flow rate in the presence of a detrusor contraction of adequate force, duration, and speed" [7].

3.4.3   Cystoscopic Image(s)

3.4.4   Suggested Treatments

Determination of treatment is typically made based upon the severity of symptoms when no absolute indications for surgery are present. Stratifying symptoms into mild, moderate, and severe can be performed by utilizing the AUA symptom score and/or the International Prostate Symptom Score (IPSS). It should be noted, however, that these symptom scores assessments are not specific to BPH but rather assess the severity of voiding symptoms.

Initial management of BPH with mild voiding symptoms includes watchful waiting or consideration of pharmacological therapy. Watchful waiting is appropriate in mild cases because only a fraction of men will have progression of symptoms or deterioration of quality of life. Pharmacologic therapy includes the prescription of alpha-adrenergic antagonists, 5 alpha reductase inhibitors, or both [6].

Absolute indications for surgery include refractory or repeat urinary retention, associated renal injury/azotemia, recurrent gross hematuria, recurrent/residual infection, bladder calculi, and large bladder diverticula; assuming the bladder remains working.

Summary Key Points
- Occurs with aging/cumulative lifelong exposure to androgens.
- Presents with obstructive symptoms.
- Diagnostics: Simple urodynamic testing: PVR and uroflowmetry.

  - Peak flow rate of less than 15 ml/s indicative of obstruction (requires adequate voided volume and curve on graph).

- *Cystoscopic appearance:* Encroachment of the prostatic urethra by the lateral and median lobes of the prostate. Visualization of the bladder's lumen with the scope resting at the veru is obscured due to the hypertrophy of the gland (see Figs. 3.14, 3.15, and 3.16).
- Treatment: watchful waiting, versus conservative therapy, versus surgical interventions.

  - AUA symptom score and/or the IPSS may be used to help stratify patients for treatment.
  - Absolute indications for surgery: refractory or repeat urinary retention, associated renal injury/azotemia, recurrent gross hematuria, recurrent/residual infection, bladder calculi, and large bladder diverticula.

Fig. 3.14 Pictured is retroflex cystoscopic assessment of the bladder neck. The large protruding mass is an obstructing median lobe protruding into the bladder with enlarged varices

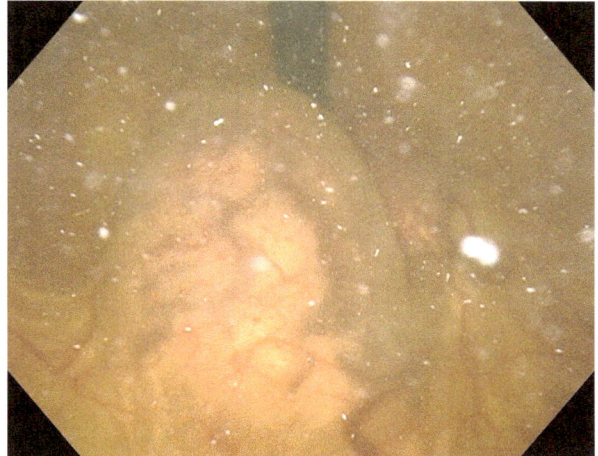

Fig. 3.15 Obstructing lateral "kissing" lobes of a prostatic urethra. This patient had significant obstructive lower urinary tract symptoms

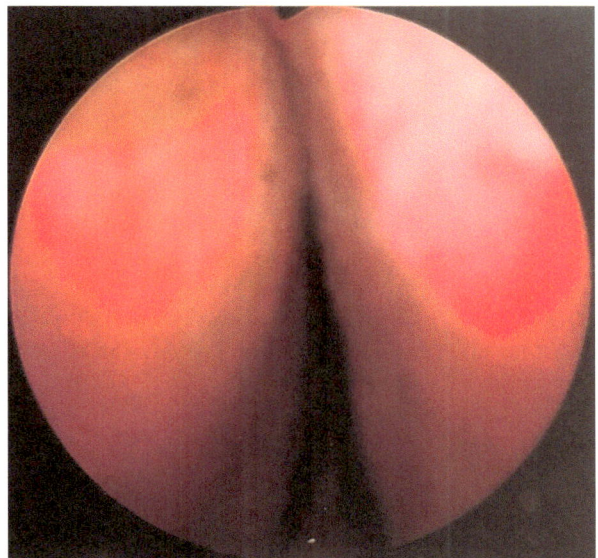

Additional References for Consideration

- Penn Clinical Manual of Urology by Philip M. Hanno MD, MPH, Thomas J. Guzzo MD, MPH, S. Bruce Malkowicz MD and Alan J. Wein MD, FACS, PhD
- Campbell-Walsh-Wein Urology by Alan W. Partin MD, PhD, Roger R. Dmochowski D, MMHC, FACS, Louis R. Kavoussi MD, MBA, and Craig A. Peters M

Fig. 3.16 The bladder neck and lumen coming into visualization. The base of the bladder is noted to be obscured by a prominent median lobe and high bladder neck

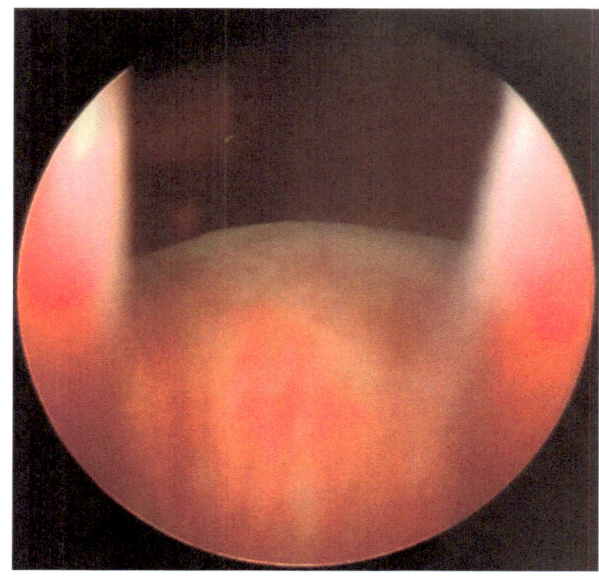

3.5   Prostate Abscess/Infection

Acute prostatitis is rarely encountered on diagnostic cystoscopy, and the introduction of a scope into an infected urinary tract should cautiously be performed only by an experienced cystoscopist. For instance, a clinician may perform cystourethroscopy in order to unroof, incise, a prostatic abscess if a patient is clinically toxic (see Figs. 3.17, 3.18, and 3.19). He or she, may also have to get emergent urinary drainage in an obstructed system with a resultant prostatic infection. Due to this, we will only briefly cover this topic.

3.5.1   Pathophysiology

Prostatitis is an infection or inflammatory process of the prostate. Infection is common in patients who have a past medical history of immunodeficiency, uncontrolled diabetes, bladder outlet obstruction, or in those who have untreated/ inadequately treated prostatitis. The most common implicated organisms are

Fig. 3.17 Transurethral
resection of prostatic
abscess

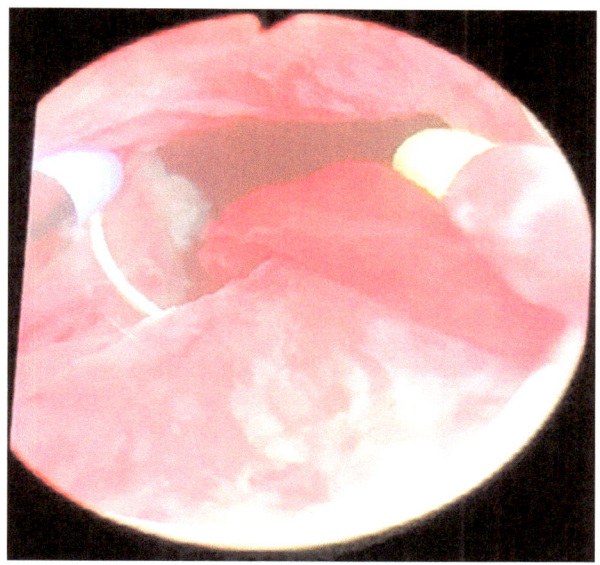

uropathogens that cause infection by ascending the male urethra. However, the
infection of *Staphylococcus aureus* should warrant the consideration of possible
hematogenous spread.

3.5.2 Clinical Presentation

Patients will typically present toxic, endorsing fevers and chills. Vital signs will cor-
roborate clinically reported symptoms with an elevated temperature. Patients will
additionally experience dysuria and obstructive voiding symptoms from prostate
edema. Laboratory workup will demonstrate leukocytosis, likely with left shift, and
computed tomography with IV contrast will likely characterize the lesion for operative planning. Transrectal ultrasound (US) is an additional viable option and can
offer co-occurring drainage via needle aspiration, if the lesion is found within the
periphery of the gland.

Fig. 3.18 Transurethral
resection of prostate
abscess with immediate
expulsion of pus

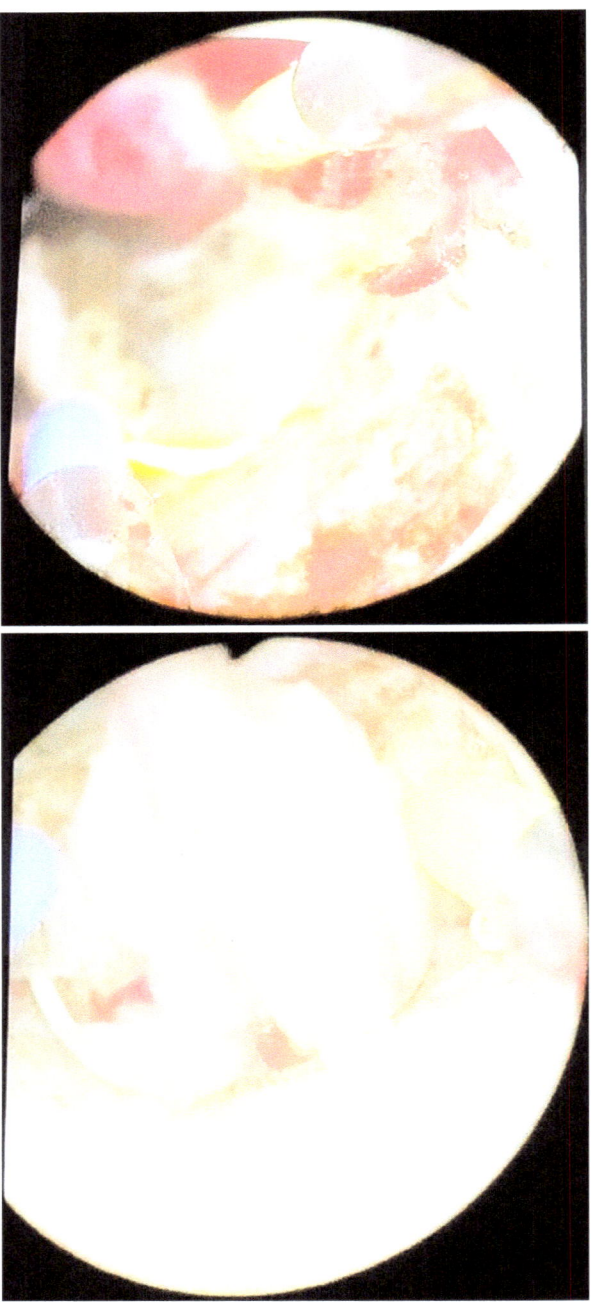

Fig. 3.19 Transurethral resection of prostate abscess with immediate expulsion of pus

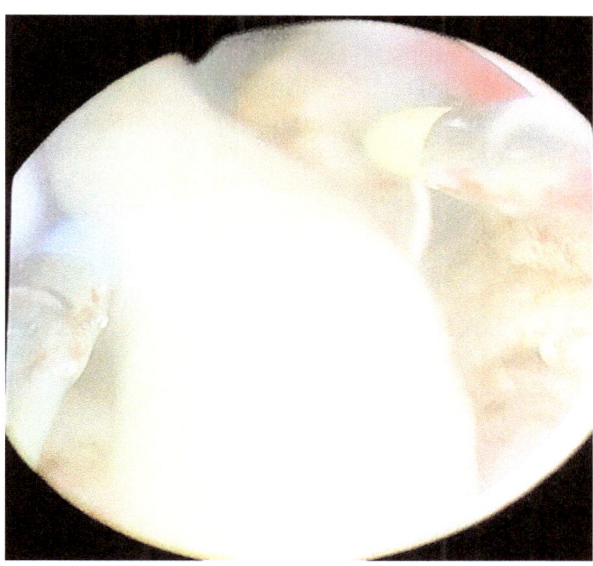

3.5.3   Cystoscopic Image(s)

3.5.4   Suggested Treatments

Abscess treatment typically requires incision/aspiration and drainage. Small abscess, less than 2 cm, may resolve with antibiotic therapy alone. Antibiotic duration is typically 4–6 weeks. Drainage via the transurethral route is favored when the abscess has a centralized location within the gland, suggesting a proximal location the urethra. Transrectal US-guided aspiration can have a reoccurrence rate of 15–33% [8].

Summary Key Points
- Infection primarily secondary to ascending urethral pathogens. Staphylococcus should warrant consideration of hematogenous spread.
- Patients will likely exhibit systemic signs and symptoms of infection (fever, chills, malaise). There may also be reports of urinary retention, dysuria, and/or perineal discomfort.
- Diagnostics: CBC to assess severity of systemic illness/infection. CT scan, with contrast, preferred test for diagnosing prostate abscess.
- *Cystoscopic appearance:* Prostate gland may appear normal or may have a prominent lobe indicating involvement.

  – Cystoscopy should only be performed while planning to intervene/unroof the abscess. Unnecessary stimulation of the infected prostate can result in hematogenous spread of bacteria.

- Treatment: Antibiotics, typically will receive initial IV with transition to PO. Duration 4–6 weeks. Large abscess, >2 cm, will likely require procedure for primary drainage of the abscess.

Additional References for Consideration
- Penn Clinical Manual of Urology by Philip M. Hanno MD, MPH, Thomas J. Guzzo MD, MPH, S. Bruce Malkowicz MD, and Alan J. Wein MD, FACS, PhD.
- Campbell-Walsh-Wein Urology by Alan W. Partin MD, Ph, Roger R. Dmochowski D, MMHC, FACS, Louis R. Kavoussi MD, MBA, and Craig A. Peters M.
- Mandell, Douglas, and Bennett's Principles and Practice of Infectious Diseases, ii-ii, by John E. Bennet MD, Raphael Dolin MD, and Martin J. Blaser MD.

3.6   Urethral Diverticulum and Urethral Fistula

3.6.1   Pathophysiology

A diverticulum is an outpouching of a hollow structure within the human body. Diverticulums can occur anywhere along the GU tract with a preponderance in the bladder and the urethra. In the female patient, most diverticulum are acquired due to paraurethral/Skene's gland infection or inflammation leading to cystic dilation. The cystic dilation will progress leading to herniation of the cystic sac transmurally through the urethra. Implicated organisms include gonococcus and, interestingly, normal vaginal flora colonization of the urethra. The incidence of urethral diverticula is approx. 1–5% with a peak prevalence around the third and fifth decade of life, and lastly with a female predilection [9].

A fistula is defined as an abnormal connection between any two hollow structures within the human body. As such, a urethra fistula is a connection between the male or female urethra to an adjacent hollow structure. Urethra fistulas predominantly occur in females resulting in a urethrovaginal fistula; however, rectourethral fistulas do occur in men. In the industrialized world, most urethral fistula formations are iatrogenic in comparison to the emerging world being secondary to parturition/prolonged labor. Other causes include congenital anomalies, malignancy, ischemia, chronic inflammation, and infection.

Urethrovaginal fistulas, as previously mentioned, are usually secondary to post-surgical complications from procedures such as urethral diverticulectomy and anti-incontinence surgery. Generally, the organ affected is where the prior surgery had taken place.

Acquired rectourethral fistula (RUF) is the predominant urethral fistulous formation in males. It can occur following prostatectomy, external beam radiotherapy, pelvic brachytherapy, and of course following trauma or inflammatory diseases of the pelvis (for example, Chron's disease or abscess). Iatrogenic injury is the leading cause of this problem, however the incidence is quire rate; the reported incidence of rectal injury following prostatectomy is only approx. 1–2%, and not all rectal injuries will result in fistula formation [10].

3.6.2   Clinical Presentation

The urethral diverticulum is best assessed upon retraction of the scope from the bladder out of the urethra. This allows for better distention in comparison to when the camera is initially inserted retrograde into the patient. If the urethral diverticulum is wide, it may accommodate the cystoscope. The cystoscopist should pay close attention to the floor and side walls of the urethra for identification of the diverticulum os (see Figs. 3.20 and 3.21). Once identified, vaginoscopy or pelvic exam should be performed to assess the diverticulum's expanse from the contralateral side. On vaginoscopy there will be an anterior vaginal wall mass. Palpation or compression of the mass via cystoscope can lead to evacuation of purulent urine or secretions from the diverticulum back within the GU tract.

Patients will typically present with a complaint of dysuria, dyspareunia, and dribbling post void. In fact, this triad used to be called the "three D's"; however, it has been found that only 5% of patients with UD will have all three complaints [11]. Recurrent UTIs are common and likely contribute to the above symptomatology and should always warrant consideration for genitourinary imaging or cystoscopic evaluation.

Symptomatology from a fistula will depend on the location of involvement. In women whose fistula occurs within the distal third of the urethra they will generally not experience any incontinence, as the opening is not proximal to the striated sphincter. There may, however, be reports of recurrent urinary tract or vaginal infections. Fistulous tracts that occur within the proximal urethra will have persistent incontinence secondary to near-immediate efflux of stored urine from the bladder into the vaginal vault.

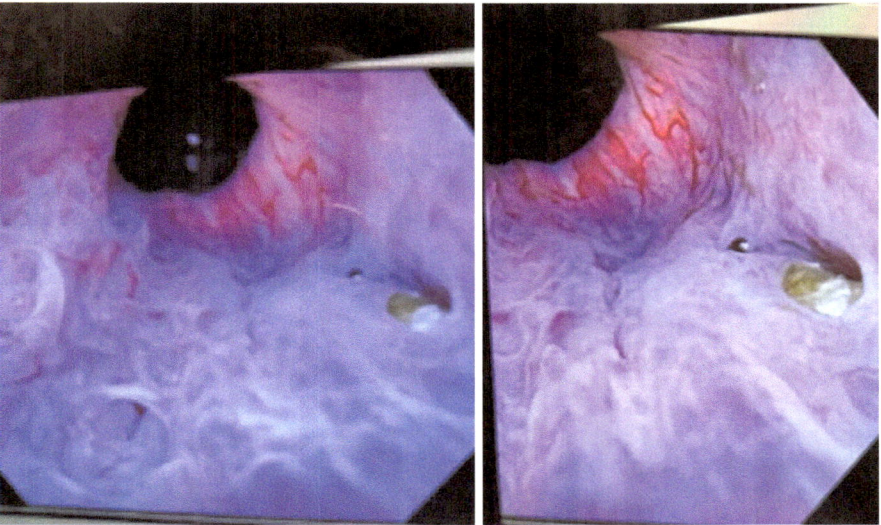

Fig. 3.20 Patient with two small diverticula sacs pictured above, located at 7 and 3 o'clock. One os is seen with a protruding small stone, and the other more inferior lateral. Narrow band imaging was used to assess the surrounding mucosa given the risk of malignancy

Fig. 3.21 Close-up of the
small lateral diverticular os

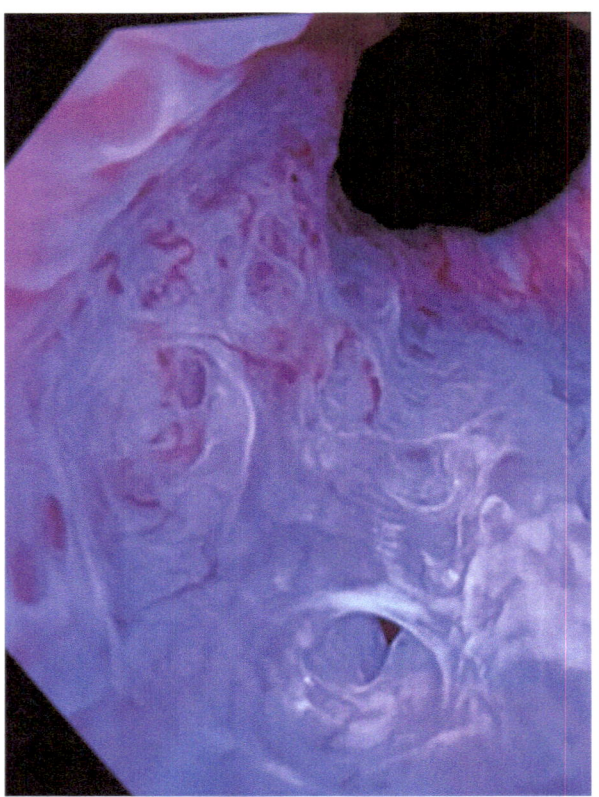

Diagnosis of a urethrovaginal fistula is made upon visualization of the fistulous tract on cystourethroscopy or voiding cystourethrogram. For radiographic examination to be sufficient, the patient must have competent sphincter at baseline as the leakage of contrast will alternatively be urethral.

Patients who have an acquired rectourethral fistula will typically present in the outpatient setting with recurrent UTI, fecaluria, pneumaturia, or possibly pain in the rectum. Diagnosis is made by voiding cystourethroscopy, cystourethroscopy and/or colonoscopy, and lastly CT or MRI to help rule in etiology.

3.6.3   Cystoscopic Image(s)

The orifice entering a urethral fistulous tract will appear similar to the ostium found with a urethral diverticulum. If the fistula's os is large in size, there may be an inability to distend the urethra with noted efflux of irrigant out of the vagina or rectum. Please see the figures provided in the urethral diverticulum section for reference.

3.6.4 Suggested Treatments

Diverticulum sacs should be inspected under direct visualization, if possible, when encountering no stenosed os/sinus, due to a risk of malignant tumor formation. Malignant tumors of adenocarcinoma, squamous cell, and transition cell carcinoma are known to occur due to the chronic inflammation that causes these diverticula.

Diverticulums can also have stones secondary to urinary stasis leading to precipitation of urinary crystals. Reported incidence of stone formation is around 1.5–10% [9]. Treatment can consist of endoscopic incision of urethral diverticulum sinus to evacuate pus (saucerization = multiple incisions), intra-diverticular lithotripsy, and open surgery.

Surgery is the preferred treatment of choice; once the diverticulum has epithelialized with the urethral lumen, conservative management with antibiotics is unsuccessful in repairing the anatomic defect. Surgery involves excision of the diverticulum with repair of the urethra.

Treatment for fistula will vary slightly contingent upon the organs involved; however, it will predominantly require surgery. In urethrovaginal fistula patients' catheter drainage has limited use, as once the tract has epithelialized the likelihood of spontaneous regression decreases exponentially. Transvaginal surgical excision with reconstruction using a flap, transposed tissue for support, is the definitive treatment option.

Treatment of a rectourethral fistula is usually performed in a two-stage approach with fecal diversion via colostomy to allow control of the continued inflammatory process. Urethral catheter drainage is also implicated in an attempt to maximally drain the bladder and prevent continued fistulous drainage. Surgical repair can include multiple approaches dependent upon the primary leading surgical team (abdominal, perineal, and/or transrectally). As in, the urethrovaginal fistula repair transposition of a flap reduces the likelihood of reoccurrence post-surgery.

Summary Key Points
Urethral Diverticulum

- Female predominance, with etiology secondary to Skene's gland infection or inflammation leading to cystic dilation.

    - Incidence 1–5% with peak prevalence around 30–50 years of age.

- Patient may present with recurrent urinary tract infection.

    - "Three D's"- dysuria, dyspareunia, and dribbling post void (5% will have all three symptoms simultaneously)

- Diagnosed via cystoscopy and radiographic imaging.

    - Double balloon PPU study and/or MRI.

- *Cystoscopic appearance:* Diverticular os can range in size and shape; can be difficult to detect. The ostium is often located low laterally at the 4 and 8 o'clock positions and at level of the mid-urethra (see Fig. 3.22).
- Treatment can consist of multiple endoscopic incisions of urethral diverticulum sinus to intra-diverticular lithotripsy, and open surgery.

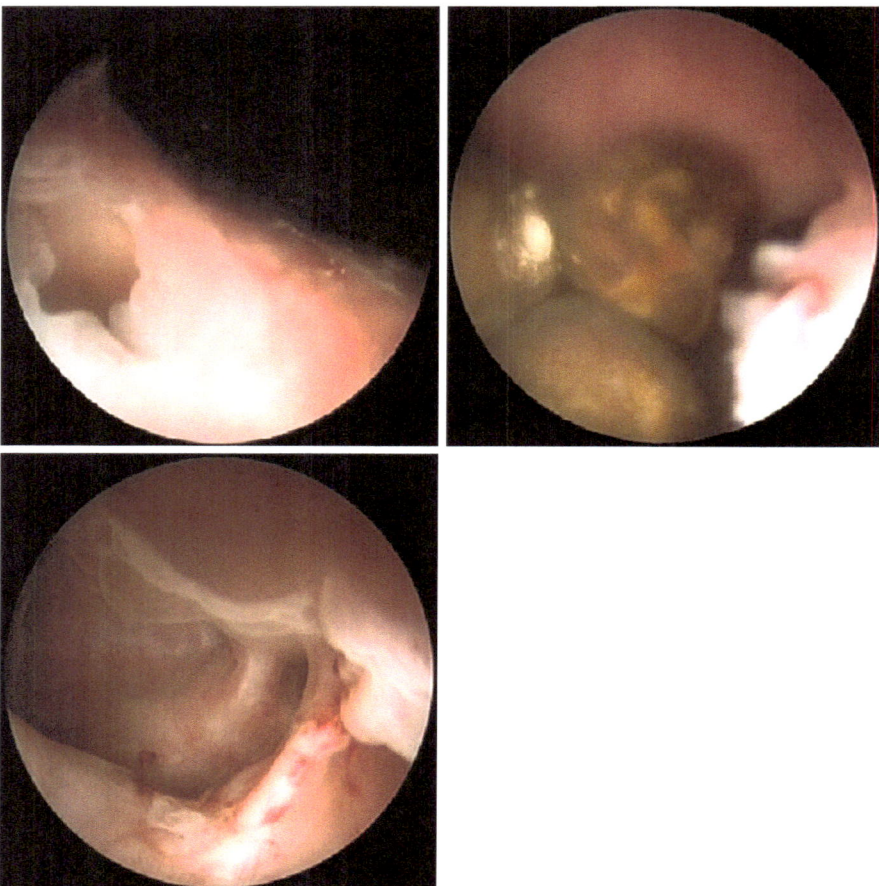

Fig. 3.22 The above three photos are provided by Dr. Gadimaliyev, who published a case report of a urethral diverticulum calculi in a male patient. Per cystoscopic examination there was identified a diverticular os on the bladder neck/posterior urthera. Further investigation of the diverticular sac demonstrated multiple triangular-shaped stones. The last image was taken following removal using a flexible grasper through the nephroscope [12]

– Surgical excision of the sac is the preferred treatment of choice once the diverticular sac has epithelialized.

Urethral Fistula

• A fistula can develop secondary to chronic inflammation or acute ischemia injury. Female predominance, with most common being urethrovaginal but can develop along the whole urinary tract.

  – Male fistulas tend to be acquired rectourethral fistulas that develop as a complication to radiation or surgery (remains rare, 1–2% of rectal injuries).

- Symptomatology dependent upon the location within the urethra (above or below the continent sphincter) and related to the involved organs.
- Diagnosis is made by voiding cystourethroscopy, cystourethroscopy and/or colonoscopy, and lastly CT or MRI to help rule in etiology.
- *Cystoscopic appearance:* The os to the urethral fistula tends to appear similar to the os found with urethral diverticular disease. Large ostium that can accommodate the scope may be traversed to assess the extent to the other organs involved.
- Treatment: Predominantly requires surgery. Small acute fistulas may resolve with catheter placement/urine diversion; however, the likelihood of spontaneous regress decreases exponentially the longer the duration and larger the fistula is.

Additional References for Consideration
- Endoscopic Diagnosis and Treatment in Urethral Pathology by Geavlete, Petrisor A.
- Campbell-Walsh-Wein Urology by Alan W. Partin MD, PhD, Roger R. Dmochowski D, MMHC, FACS, Louis R. Kavoussi MD, MBA, and Craig A. Peters M.
- Penn Clinical Manual of Urology by Philip M. Hanno MD, MPH, Thomas J. Guzzo MD, MPH, S. Bruce Malkowicz MD, and Alan J. Wein MD, FACS, PhD.
- Endoscopic Diagnosis and Treatment in Urethral Pathology by Geavlete, Petrisor A.

3.7 Urethral Tumors (Benign)

3.7.1 Pathophysiology

Benign urethral tumors can be divided into the following categories based upon the cell layer of involvement or etiology: epithelial/mixed tumors, mesenchymal tumors, and inflammatory (False) polyps. These tumors occur throughout the urethra, with a reported greater incidence of polyp formation within the prostatic urethra in men [9].

False polyps occur due to inflammation causing granulation of the urothelium (see Figs. 3.23 and 3.24). These lesions may represent the initial stage in the development of acquired fibroepithelial polyps, on the outer skin surface these are termed skin tags (see Figs. 3.25 and 3.26). This can also occur along the urothelium in the setting of chronic inflammation. Other false polyps include villous polyps that occur along the verumontanum around the fourth decade of life, and inverted papillomas.

Mesenchymal tumors include hemangiomas, fibromas, or myomas, as these arise from the supportive/connective tissue. Differentiation of type of tumor is primarily only made by microscopic/histologic identification. There are, however, certain features of a tumor or polyp that would suggest a more benign pathology. Benign lesions may appear translucent or similar in appearance to the surrounding mucosa; in these cases, there is less local inflammation surrounding the tumor.

Fig. 3.23 False polyp; benign appearing urethral polyp proximal to a pendulous urethral stricture. Note the uniform appearance to the surrounding mucosa

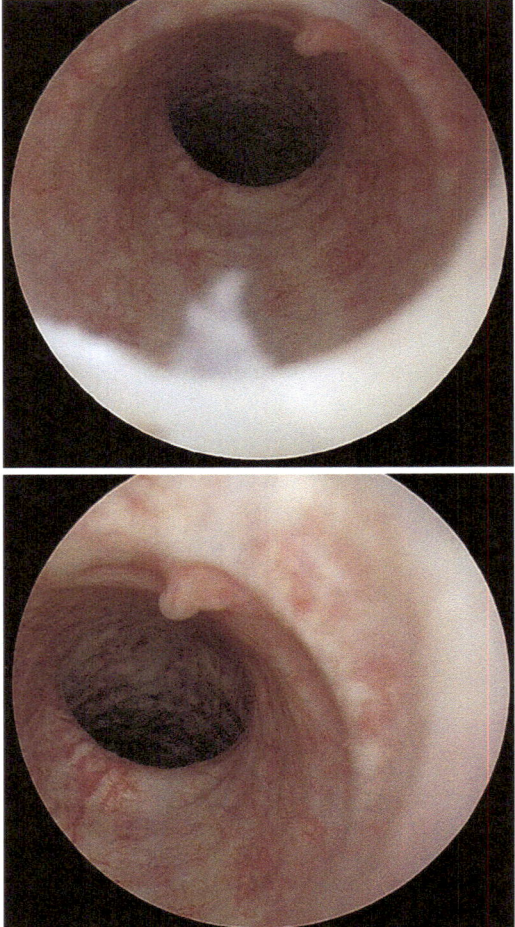

Fig. 3.24 Status post biopsy of the urethral lesion. Histologic examination revealed benign polypoid urethral tissue

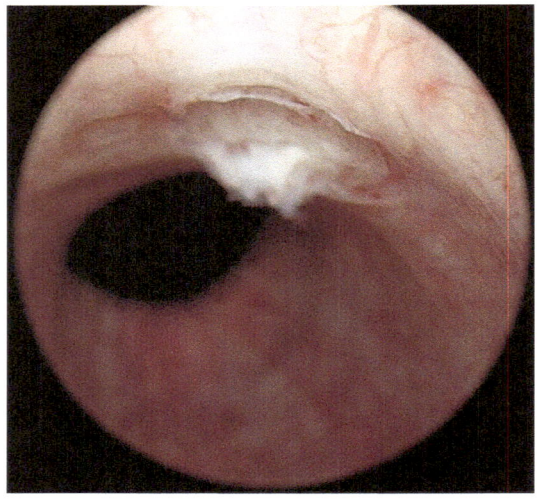

Fig. 3.25 Large fibroepithelial polyp extending into the bladder neck and implanted on the dorsal plane of the veru. Patient had reported obstructive symptoms warranting cystoscopy with TUR

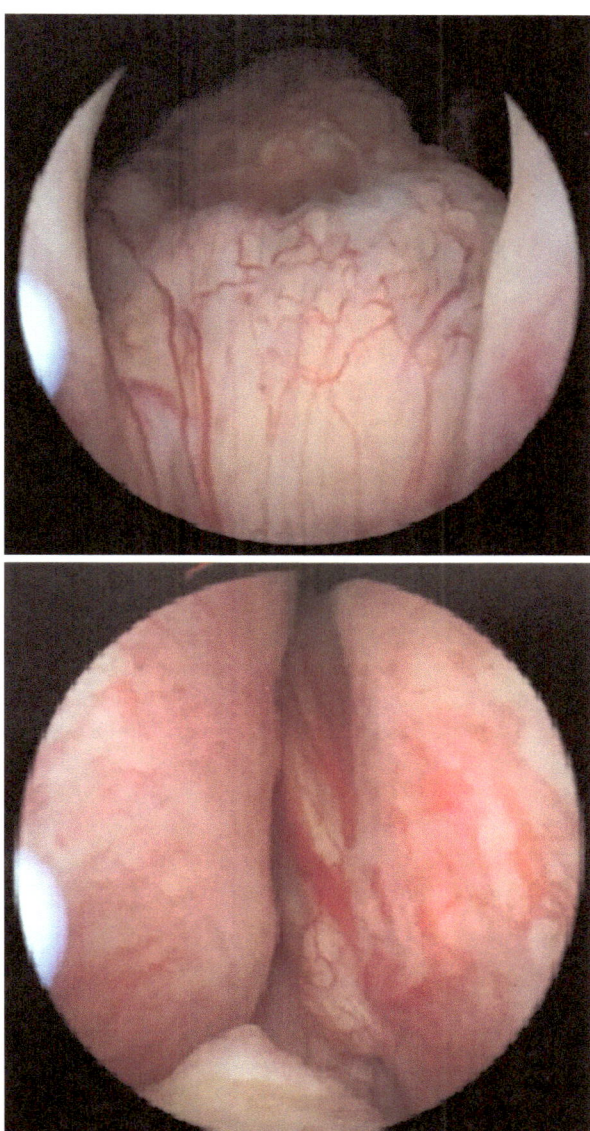

Other categorically different urethral tumors include those that arise from viruses, such as condyloma acuminata due to human papillomavirus family. Urethral condylomas occur due to direct seeding of noninfected basal epithelial cells by their infected neighbors. This then makes sense that these lesions typically result in the distal posterior urethra.

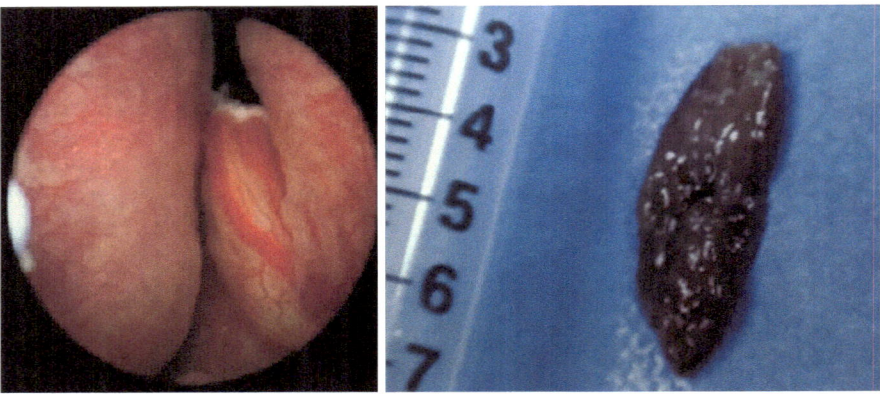

Fig. 3.26 Upon resection of the benign fibroepithelial tumor it was measuring 2–2.5 cm. Photos of the fibroepithelial tumor were provided thanks to Dr. Mark Makhuli at Atrium Health Hospital

3.7.2   Clinical Presentation

Patients with benign urethra tumors may be asymptomatic or present with symptoms of outlet obstruction if the lesion is large enough to occupy most of the urethral lumen. He or she may have decreased urinary stream, dribbling, high pressure voiding, dysuria, and possible hematuria. They may also complain of a visible lesion, as in those with a urethra caruncle or condyloma acuminata. If a genital wart is found, the urethral meatus should be inspected by gentle retraction in order to ensure no meatal lesion is present. If there is a lesion present, cystourethroscopy should be performed to assess the extent of urethral involvement, but it is recommended that a gauze dressing be wrapped tightly around the base of the penis to prevent seeding of the anterior urethra, or urethroscopy stopped in front of the striated sphincter.

3.7.3   Cystoscopic Image(s)

3.7.4   Suggested Treatments

Diagnostic urethroscopy assists in identifying the tumor: characterizing the number, location, and appearance. It may also allow for biopsy using a cold-cup flexible biopsy forceps, but care should be taken when performing this, as electrocauterization may be required if extensive hematuria were to develop.

Benign urethral tumors can be treated endoscopically, unless treating for a urethral caruncle where surgical excision is preferred due to its distal location. Hemangiomas may spontaneously regress if small, but larger lesions require endoscopic resection and electrofulguration as these will bleed. Condylomas are known to reoccur approx. 21–47% of the time when treated endoscopically, with the lower incidence attributed to improved photodynamic diagnosis and ablation with a Nd:YAG laser [2].

Summary Key Points

- Benign urethral tumor types: Epithelial/mixed tumors, mesenchymal tumors, and inflammatory/false polyps.
- Condition can have symptoms ranging from asymptomatic, associated UTI symptoms, obstructive symptoms secondary to blocking mass, etc.
- Diagnosis made on cystoscopy.
- *Cystoscopic appearance:* Tumor appearance can vary from small polyps with a normal appearing mucosa to more erythematous lesions. Biopsy is the only way to truly differentiate benign versus malignant pathology.

  – Benign lesions may appear translucent or similar in appearance to the surrounding mucosa.

- Treatment: Biopsy with electrocauterization successfully treats benign lesions. Small lesions may involute spontaneously. Tumors secondary to Condyloma are commonly ablated with Nd:YAG laser.

Additional References for Consideration

- Penn Clinical Manual of Urology by Philip M. Hanno MD, MPH, Thomas J. Guzzo MD, MPH, S. Bruce Malkowicz MD, and Alan J. Wein MD, FACS, PhD.
- Endoscopic Diagnosis and Treatment in Urethral Pathology by Geavlete, Petrisor A.

3.8 Urethral Trauma

3.8.1 Pathophysiology

Trauma resulting from unintentional injuries is the leading cause of death for patients aged 45 and younger [13]. The lower urinary tract is susceptible to injury with urethral injuries categorized by the location of insult, either posterior or anterior urethral injuries. Posterior urethral injuries tend to result from an anterior pelvic ring fracture or pubic diastasis. In fact, urethral injuries occur in up to 10% of males and 6% of females with pelvic factures [14]. Straddle fractures are arguably the worst variety of pelvic fractures with all four pubic rami being involved resulting in near guarantee of urologic injury [15]. The mechanism of urethral disruption with posterior urethral injuries is due to the fixed location of the posterior urethra, which includes the membranous urethra and the prostate, to the pubis via puboprostatic ligaments. When a shearing force causes an opposite movement of the prostate from the membranous urethra the result is a urethral defect, tear, or disruption at this location.

Anterior urethral injuries differ from posterior urethral injuries in that the mechanism of injury is primarily secondary to compression, as the bulbar urethra sandwiches under the pubis [16]. This injury is primarily termed a "straddle injury". The most common morbidity of a straddle injury is urethral stricture disease [17].

3.8.2   Clinical Presentation

Presentation of said patients is usually made by initial consultation by the trauma service. This may occur due to an inability to insert a Foley catheter, or the correct caution that comes with blood at the urethral meatus. When consulted, the urology clinician should heavily suspect a urethral disruption in any patient who has had a pelvic fracture with an inability to urinate, blood at the meatus, and a palpably full bladder.

When blood is visible at the male urethral meatus, an immediate retrograde urethrogram should be performed to rule out the finding of urethral disruption [18]. This is performed at bedside using a portable c-arm x-ray machine. In a female patient, direct cystoscopic inspection is warranted (see Fig. 3.27).

Fig. 3.27 Urethral erosion (mild above and severe below) within the pendulous urethra secondary to forceful Foley catheter attempt in the setting of urethral stricture disease

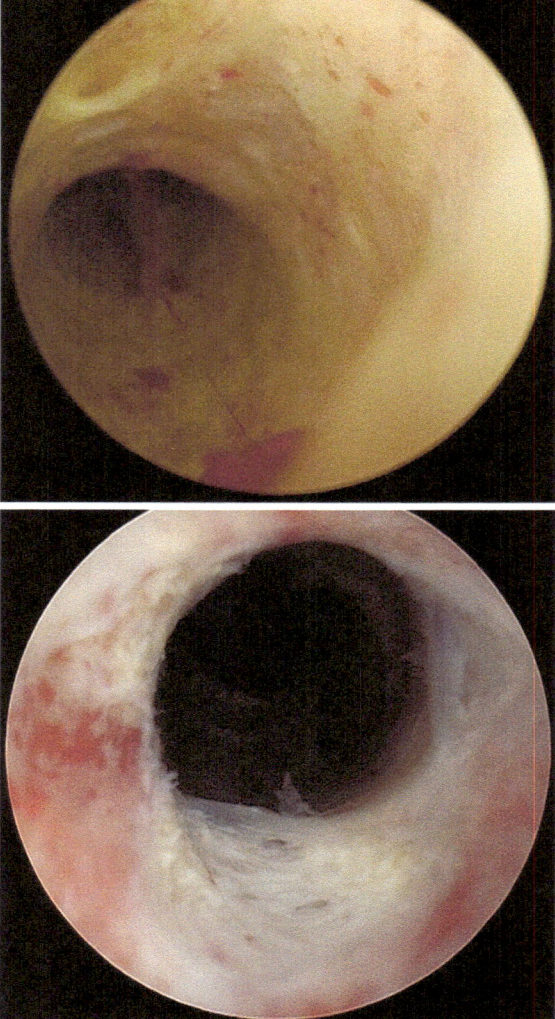

3.8.3   Cystoscopic Image(s)

3.8.4   Suggested Treatments

Initial management of a urethral injury has two suggested courses: (1) insertion of a suprapubic cystostomy with planned delayed reconstruction, or (2) primary realignment with urethral Foley catheter insertion. Primary realignment attempts should be brief in duration given the risk of infection for prolonged procedures. After primary realignment, the catheter should remain either 4–6 weeks, prior to permanent removal either a diagnostic cystourethroscopy should be performed or repeat retrograde urethrograms to ensure the wound has scared down/healed.

Delayed reconstruction, after primary bladder drainage using a suprapubic cystostomy, occurs 2–3 months post injury after the scar has fully matured. Preoperative evaluation for these procedures includes a cystogram (voided attempt) and retrograde urethrogram (colloquially called "up-and-down-o-gram") in order to assess the length of the matured scar.

Summary Key Points
- Anterior urethral injuries occur secondary to compression of the bulbar urethra under the pubis. Posterior urethral injuries tend to result from an anterior pelvic ring fracture or pubic diastasis.

  – Straddle fracture- all four pubic rami fractured, nearly guaranteeing urethral involvement.

- Patients who present following a known trauma to the pelvis may have co-occurring urinary retention, bloody urethral discharge, and frank injury or bruising to the external genitalia.
- Diagnosis: Recommended to perform an immediate retrograde urethrogram when blood is appreciated at the urethral meatus (AUA guidelines).

  – CT scan and pelvic x rays will assist in diagnosis.

- *Cystoscopic appearance:* Urethral trauma can range from urethral erosion of the mucosa to complete avulsion/disruption. The true lumen of the urethra typically takes an anterior route when there is a fork on urethroscopy 2/2 to a false passage.
- Treatment: SPT insertion with planned delayed reconstruction versus primary realignment.

  – Primary realignment attempts should be brief. If there is success with a true disruption the catheter should remain for 4–6 weeks. Cystoscopy can be repeated at the time of removal to assess for either stricture disease and adequate wound healing.

Additional References for Consideration
- Campbell-Walsh-Wein Urology by Alan W. Partin MD, PhD, Roger R. Dmochowski D, MMHC, FACS, Louis R. Kavoussi MD, MBA, and Craig A. Peters M Urinary Fistula, 2014)

3.9 Medical Devices/Artificial Urinary Sphincter

3.9.1 Pathophysiology

Urinary incontinence is best summarized as involuntary, accidental, loss of urine that is secondary to either outlet abnormalities, bladder abnormalities, or both. The international continence society defines stress urinary incontinence as "the complaint of any involuntary loss of urine on effort or physical exertion or on sneezing or coughing" [19]. Stress incontinence thus is attributed to episodes of increased intra-abdominal pressure that then overcome outlet resistance, again due to either bladder or outlet abnormalities. Urge incontinence is differentiated from stress incontinence by symptomatology, or the report incontinence upon the sense of needing to urinate during a bladder contraction.

In males, due to the presence of two anatomical sphincters within the urethra, there must be concomitant impairment of the internal (bladder neck and prostate) and external sphincter (rhabdosphincter) for incontinence to occur. This is likely why male incontinence is only about 5–6% of the general geriatric population [20].

3.9.2 Clinical Presentation

Artificial urinary sphincters are employed for patients who have sphincteric incontinence. In general, a single cuff/artificial sphincter perineal approach is preferred. The goal during surgery is to place the cuff as proximal on the bulbar urethra as possible. Outcomes for the surgery are good with at least 89% of patients endorsing some form of improvement and 75% endorsing cure [20].

Possible complications from artificial urinary sphincter insertion do occur albeit are not common. The clinician who finds themselves encountering a person with an undisclosed history of urologic surgery and presenting with urinary retention should have a malfunctioning AUS within the differential. Urethral erosion can also occur, and it has a reported incidence of around 5–10%. Device longevity has an expectation of approx. 10 years [21] (see Fig. 3.28).

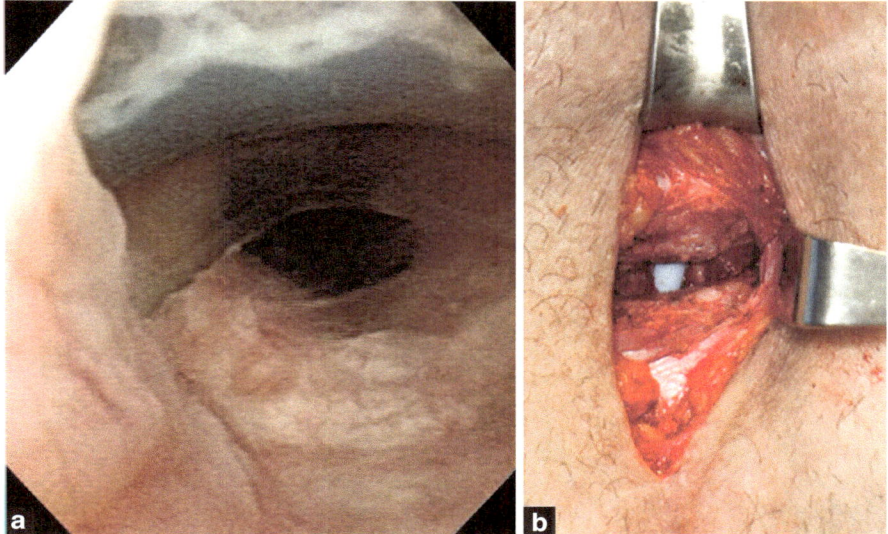

Fig. 3.28 Pictured below are both the urethroscopic assessment of an artificial urinary sphincter erosion (**a**) and the subsequent explanation with evident urethral defect as evidenced by blue wire in urethra (**b**). On the left, seen superiorly, is the balloon filled with sterile solution. Photos provided by Doctors Agarwal, Linder, and Elliot [22]

3.9.3   Cystoscopic Image(s)

Additional References for Consideration
- Surgical Treatment for Urinary Incontinence in Men by International Continence Society.
- Campbell-Walsh-Wein Urology by Alan W. Partin MD, PhD, Roger R. Dmochowski D, MMHC, FACS, Louis R. Kavoussi MD, MBA, and Craig A. Peters M.

References

1. Hanno P. Lower urinary tract infections and pyelonephritis. In: Hanno P, Guzzo T, Malkowicz B, Wein A, editors. Penn clinical manual of urology. Philadelphia: Saunders; 2014. p. 110–32.
2. Zoltan E, Cockrell R. Sexually transmitted infections. In: Hanno P, Guzzo T, Malkowicz B, Wein A, editors. Penn clinical manual of urology. Philadelphia: Saunders; 2014. p. 164–94.
3. Blaivas J, Groutz A. Bladder outlet obstruction nomogram for women with lower urinary tract symptomatology. Neurourol Urodyn. 2000;19(5):553–64.
4. Metro M. Urethral stricture disease. In: Hano P, Guzzo T, Malkowicz B, Wein A, editors. Penn clinical manual of urology. Philadelphia: Saunders; 2014. p. 284–300.
5. Pal DK, Kumar S, Ghosh B. Direct visual internal urethrotomy: is it a durable treatment option? Urol Annals. 2017;9(1):18–22. https://doi.org/10.4103/0974-7796.198835.

6. Berges R, Oelke M. Age-stratified normal values for prostate volume, PSA, maimum urinary flow rate, IPSS, and other LUTS/BPH indicators in the German male community- dwelling population aged 50 years or older. World J Urol. 2011;29(2):171–8.

7. Mock S, Dmochowski R. Benign prostatic hyperplasia and related entities. In: Hanno P, Guzzo T, Malkowicz B, Wein A, editors. Penn clinical manual of urology. Philadelphia: Elsevier; 2014. p. 462–504.

8. Ackerman A, Parameshwar P, Anger J. Diagnosis and treatment of patients with prostatic abscess in the post-antibiotic era. Int J Urol. 2018;25(2):103–10.

9. Geavlete P, Dragutescu M, Multescu R, Geavlete B. Endoscopic management of urethral abnormalities. In: Geavlete P, editor. Endoscopic diagnosis and treatment in urethral pathology. San Diego: Elsevier; 2016. p. 129–98.

10. Smith A, Rovner E. Urinary fistula. In: Hanno P, Guzzo T, Malkowicz B, Wein A, editors. Penn clinical manual of urology. Philadelphia: Saunders; 2014. p. 301–18.

11. Vasavada, S., & Kim, D. (2018, Jun 13). Urethral Diverticula Clinical Presentation. Retrieved from Medscape: https://emedicine.medscape.com/article/443296.

12. Gadimaliyev E. Urethral diverticulum calculi in a male: a case report. Case Rep Urol. 2013;2013., Article ID 437106, 2 pages https://doi.org/10.1155/2013/437106.

13. Center for Disease Control. (2021, Feb 11). *Injury Prevention & Control*. Retrieved from Centers for disease control: cdc.gov/injury/wisqars/animated-leading-causes.html

14. Koraitim. Pelvic facture urethral injuries: the unresolved controversy. J Urol. 1999;161(5): 1433–41.

15. Brandes S, Borelli J. Pelvic fracture and associated urologic injuries. World Journal of Surg. 2001;25(12):1578–87.

16. Morey A, Simhan J. Genital and lower urinary tract trauma. In: Partin A, Dmochowski R, Kavoussi L, Peters C, editors. Campbell-Walsh-Wein urology. Philadelphia: Elsevier; 2021. p. 3084–61.

17. Park S, McAninch J. Straddle injuries to the bulbar urethra: management and outcomes in 78 patients. J Urol. 2004:722–5.

18. American Urology Association. (2021). *Urotrauma Guidelines*. Retrieved from AUA.NET: auanet.org/guidelines/guidelines/urotrauma-guideline#3268

19. International Continence Society. (2018, Jan 1). Stress Urinary Incontinence. Retrieved from Internatinoal Continence Society: https://www.ics.org.

20. Wessells H, Vanni A. Surgical procedures for sphincter incontinence in the male. In: Partin A, Dmochowski R, Kavoussi L, Peters C, editors. Campbell-Walsh-Wein urology. Philadelphia: Elsevier; 2021. p. 2993–3009.

21. Hoffman D, Rude T, Nitti V. Complications of surgery for male incontinence. In: Taneja S, Shah O, editors. Complications of urologic surgery. London: Elsevier; 2018. p. 535–45.

22. Elliott D, Agarwal D, Linder B, Clinic M. Artificial urinary sphincter urethral Erosinos: temporal patterns, management, and incidence of preventable erosions. Indian J Urol. 2017;33(1): 26–9.

Chapter 4
Malignant Urethral Pathology

4.1 Malignant Urethral Lesions

4.1.1 Pathophysiology

Urethral malignancy is rare, accounting for less than 1% of all genitourinary cancers (up to date urethral cancer). These tumors are either primary, arising directly from the urethra, or secondary due to metastatic invasion. The primary types of urethral cancer are thus labeled dependent upon their cell progenitor: transitional cell carcinoma, squamous cell carcinoma, adenocarcinoma, clear cell carcinoma, melanoma of the external meatus (this is a rare type of aggressive cancer), and others rare forms (small cell neuroendocrine type, plasmacytomas) [1] (see Figs. 4.1, 4.2, 4.3, and 4.4).

The most common primary histologic type found is epidermoid squamous cell carcinoma, followed by transitional cell and adenocarcinoma in males and females, respectively. Malignant tumors can arise anywhere throughout the urethra; however, there is a predilection within the bulbar-membranous segment in males (60%) [1].

Male primary urethral cancers can be grouped by location of occurrence within the urethra; anterior and posterior urethral cancers tend to have a slightly differing disease progression and cell type. If you recall, the anterior urethra has a layer of stratified squamous then pseudostratified squamous epithelial cells, extending from the meatus to the end of the bulbar urethra, and thus commonly has squamous cell carcinoma type. This differs from the transitional cell type within the posterior urethra of men, which carries a poorer prognosis. If a primary posterior urethral cancer is found within the male patient on urethroscopy, cystoscopic assessment of the bladder should also be performed.

B. C. Tenny, M. O'Neill, *Diagnostic Cystoscopy*, https://doi.org/10.1007/978-3-031-10668-2_4

Fig. 4.1 Pictured here is melanoma of the external urethral meatus and vestibule. Histologic examination demonstrated polypoid fragments of tissue containing malignant-appearing epithelioid cells with intracytoplasmic melanin pigmentation. The tumor cells are arranged in nodules in the submucosa, and only very focal mucosal involvement is seen

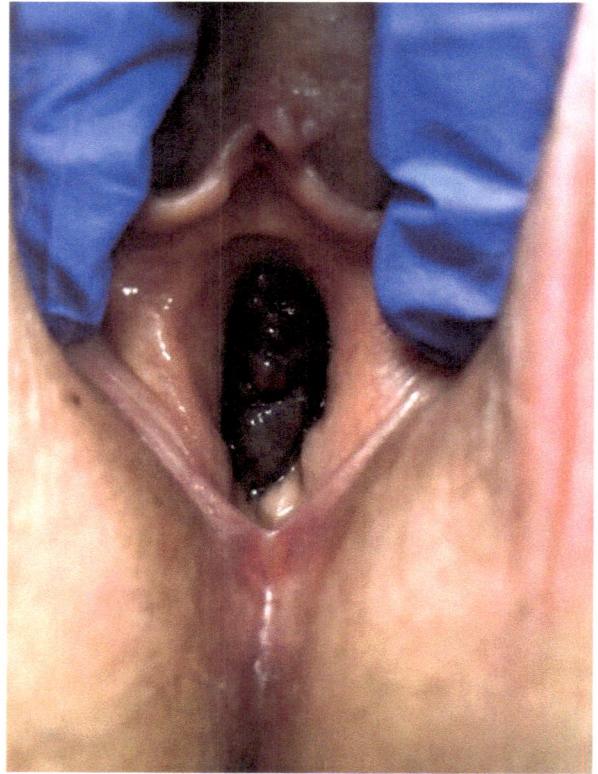

Risk factors of urethral cancer are similar to those associated with bladder cancer: prior exposure to radiotherapy, certain substances such as arsenic or heavy metals, sexually transmitted diseases, abnormal anatomy (approx. 5% of female urethral cancers occur inside a diverticula), chronic inflammation, and adjacent high-grade genitourinary cancers. For instance, urethral tumors can occur from seeding or local expansion into the urethral mucosa from primary bladder cancer (negative margins on cystectomy) [2].

Epidemiologic studies demonstrate a greater prevalence in urethral cancer in white females (four times the reported occurrence in men), and of those that do occur in men, interestingly, there is a greater incidence in black men. This greater incidence in black men among males could possibly be secondary to unequal social determinants of health, and further research should be directed with goals in increasing health parity [3].

Fig. 4.2 Pictured above is a 1 cm papillary lesion within the prostatic urethra at 8 o'clock location, just distal to bladder neck and proximal to veru. The lesion pathology confirmed TCC

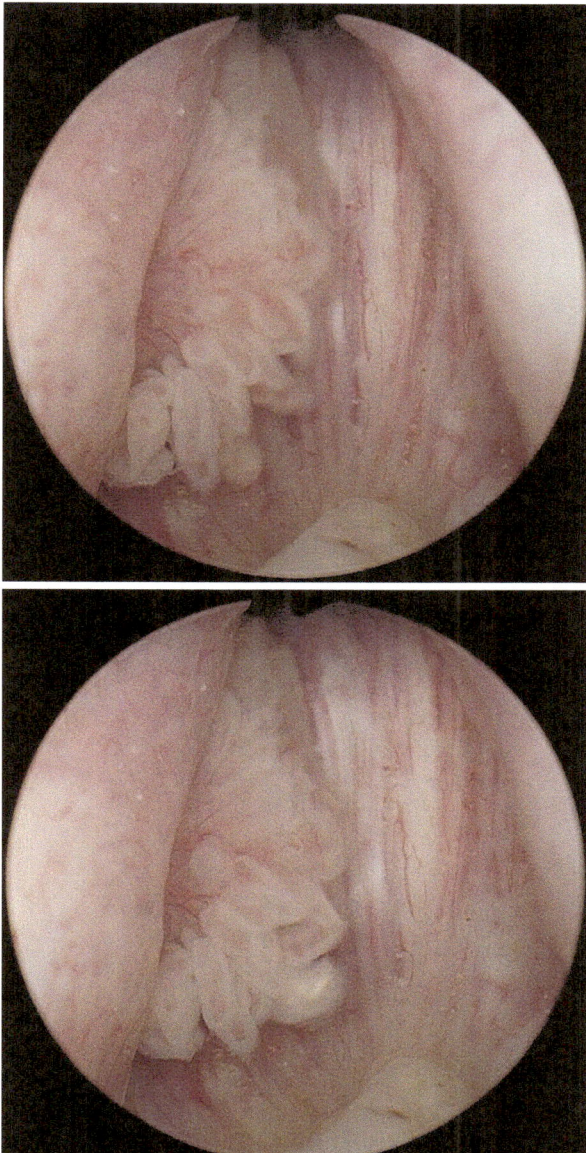

Fig. 4.3 Urothelial carcinoma lesion within the female urethra. Cancer was low grade TCC on cystoscopy biopsy

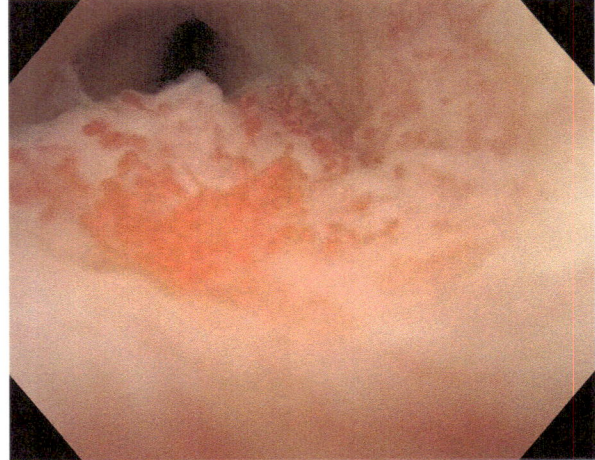

Fig. 4.4 Female bladder neck/proximal urethra with sessile papillary tumor

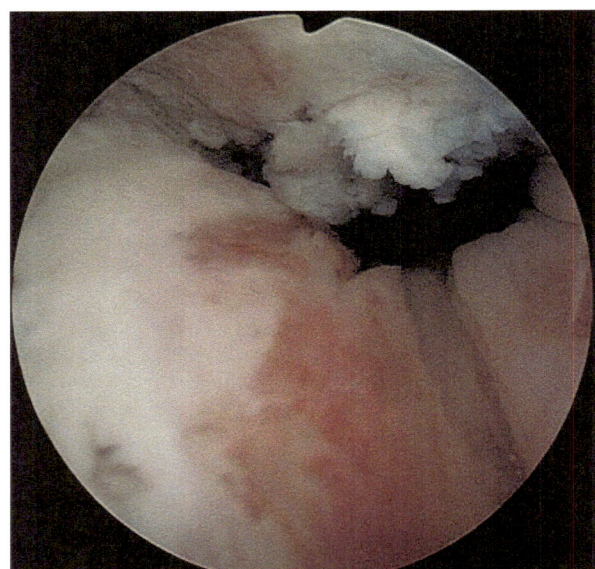

4.1.2   Clinical Presentation

One of the most common complaints or signs of genitourinary malignancy is hematuria. Hematuria can either be microscopic or gross dependent upon the degree of involvement by the tumor/lesion. Microscopic hematuria, which is found on routine urinalysis, is significant when there are >3 red blood cells (RBC) on a high power field. Red blood cells once deemed significant are then stratified by risk of having a genitourinary malignancy. Stratification of patients in low-, intermediate-, or high-risk groups are made based upon age, number of RBCs, risk factors found in urothelial cancer (smoking history, exposure to industrial dyes/solvents, etc.), multiple occurrences of microscopic hematuria, and hematuria on gross exam.

Other common complaints associated with urethral malignancy could consist of dysuria, incomplete bladder emptying, dribbling, having to strain with urination, or other lower urinary tract symptoms. Localized cancer is unlikely to have severe systemic symptoms as the cancer has not spread outside the involved organ; vice versa those that do have overt metastasis may present with extra-genitourinary complaints. Diagnosis of urethral cancer is facilitated by diagnostic cystoscopy with or without biopsy. Having tissue of the tumor allows for identification of the histologic type and further treatment planning.

4.1.3 Cystoscopic Image(s)

4.2 Suggested Treatments

Treatment of urethral tumors, similar to bladder tumors, depends upon the histologic grade/type of cancer found after biopsy, and its relative TNM scoring on diagnosis. It is important to note that recommendations for treatment, based upon the AUA guidelines are type 4 ("suggestion") rather than type 1 or 2 due to the rarity of the disease.

Biopsy of urethral lesions, if attempted upon diagnostic cystourethroscopy, uses a cold cup biopsy flexible forceps. Removal of a small tissue sample may precipitate bleeding and may be uncomfortable to the alert patient. The majority of biopsies thus occur under sedation when fulguration using a cautery/Bugbee probe can be performed.

Tumors that are superficial and well-differentiated lesions (Tis, Ta, and T1) can be treated with transurethral resection, electrofulguration, or laser ablation. These "favorable" lesions are typically found within the anterior urethra. The invasive high-grade tumors that are predominantly found within the posterior urethra typically require open surgery with radical or palliative intention [5].

Summary Key Points
- Urethral malignancy is rare, less than 1% of all GU cancers. Most common type is epidermoid squamous cell carcinoma.

  - In males there is a predilection for tumors occurring within the bulbar-membranous urethral segment. More posterior urethral lesions tend to have a grade on histologic examination.

- Signs and symptoms may include obstructive urinary symptoms from urethral lumen blockage, hematuria both gross and microscopic, and pain-associated tumor invasion.
- Diagnosis of urethral malignancy is facilitated by cystoscopy with biopsy.
- *Cystoscopic appearance:* Tumor appearance with vastly differ dependent upon the primary histologic type.
- Treatment: Superficial and low-grade tumors may be treated with resection and electrofulguration or laser ablation. High-grade tumors will likely require open surgery with radical or palliative intention.

Additional References for Consideration
- Campbell-Walsh-Wein Urology by Alan W. Partin MD, PhD, Roger R. Dmochowski D, MMHC, FACS, Louis R. Kavoussi MD, MBA, and Craig A. Peters M.

4.3   Prostate Cancer

4.3.1   Pathophysiology

Prostate cancer is the most common cancer found and the second greatest cause of cancer mortality in men [6]. In 2018, the rate of new diagnoses of prostate cancer was 107.5 in100,000 men, and the rate of prostate cancer related mortality was 18.9 per 100,000 men [7]. Prostate cancer occurs due to dysplasia of the glandular tissue of the prostate. This is thought to be secondary to mutations on genes/chromosomal rearrangements on the prostate gland causing impaired inflammatory function and/or androgen receptor dysfunction. Either way this leads to proliferation of the dysplastic cells resulting in tumor formation.

The majority of prostate cancers are adenocarcinoma type, as they develop from the acinar glands of the prostate. This occurs primarily in the peripheral zone, and much of the glandular tissue of the prostate remains in this location. If histological examination demonstrates mucin-containing glands, it is deemed a more worrisome variant. Signet ring features likewise carry a poorer prognosis.

4.3.2   Clinical Presentation

Patients with prostate cancer are typically diagnosed initially by routine prostate specific screening: digital rectal examination and serum levels of prostate-specific antigen (see Table 4.1). This has led to much of the disease being diagnosed when the patient is asymptomatic. Tumors that have loci within the central zone of the prostate may have voiding symptoms similar to the outlet obstruction seen in BPH. Screening is recommended for all men older than 55 years of age, and for men 40–54 years of age who are at higher risk for severe outcomes if cancer is present (positive family history or African American race).

Table 4.1 This table has been formatted from the AUA 2020 hematuria guidelines

Low risk: Women age < 50 years and men <40 years, never smoker or < 10 pack years, 3–10 RBCs on high power field, no risks factors for urothelial cancer, no prior episode of hematuria
Intermediate risk: Women age 50–59 and men 40–59, 10–30 pack years, 11–25 RBCs on high power field, one or more risk factors for urothelial cancer, 3–25 RBCs on prior high power field microscope exam.
High risk: Women and men >60 years, >30 RBCs on high power field, history of gross hematuria, >25 RBC on prior high power field microscope exam.

The presence of any of the above findings warrants stratification of the patient into the higher risk group [4]

4.3.2.1   AUA guidelines on PSA screening (Table 4.2)

If the PSA is elevated, the patient is then referred for a prostate biopsy. Inconclusive PSA findings can be further stratified for the likelihood of cancer by either the percentage of free PSA and the PSA density (compared to prostate gland size). Biopsy findings are then reported as a Gleason Grade in order to guide treatment recommendations. Prostate cancer found incidentally on a cystourethroscopic procedure is deemed T1a or T1b disease (determination of either "a" or "b" is contingent upon the overall percentage of neoplastic tissue on the retrieved specimen when performing a urethral prostate resection) (see Figs. 4.5 and 4.6).

Table 4.2 AUA guidelines on PSA screening

1.	PSA screening in men under the age of 40 is not recommended.
2.	Routine screening in men between the ages of 40 to 54 years at average risk is not recommended.
3.	For men 55 to 69 years old, the decision to undergo PSA screening involves weighing the benefits of preventing prostate cancer mortality in 1 man for every 1000 and screened over a decade against the known potential harms associated with screening and treatment. For this reason, shared decision-making is recommended for men age 55 to 69 years who are considering PSA screening, and proceeding based on the patient's values and preferences.
4.	To reduce the harms of screening, a routine screening interval of 2 years or more may be preferred over annual screening in those men who have participated in shared decision-making and decided on screening. As compared to annual screening, it is expected that screening intervals of 2 years preserve the majority of benefits and reduced overdiagnosis and false positives.
5.	Routine PSA screening is not recommended in any man over age 70 or any man with less than a 10 to 15 year life expectancy.

The above table has been formatted from AUA guidelines on PSA screening [8]

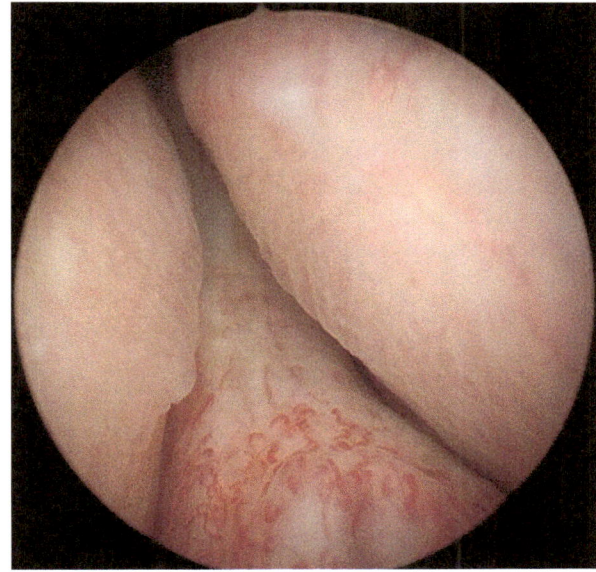

Fig. 4.5 Pictured are large obstructing lateral lobes of the prostate. Patients with prostate cancer may have obstructing lobes or a normal appearing prostatic urethra. Primarily, prostate cancer grows in the periphery of the prostate gland

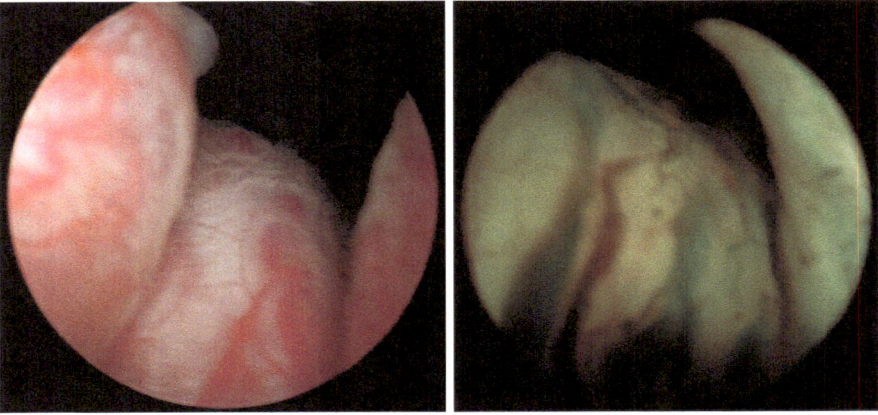

Fig. 4.6 Pre-transurethral resection of the prostate. Visualization under normal lighting and narrow band imaging. Histologic examination confirmed T1a staging

4.3.3   Cystoscopic Image(s)

4.3.4   Suggested Treatments

Treatment for prostate cancer has improved greatly over the last few decades. With the advent of robotic surgery and the ability to provide localized radiation therapy, the mortality of the disease is decreasing along with the morbidity of the medical interventions. Treatment is based upon risk stratification and the AUA guidelines go into significant detail on what treatment should be considered.

Summary Key Points
- Occurs secondary to dysplasia of the glandular tissue of the prostate.

  – Prostate cancer is the second greatest cause of cancer mortality in men.

- Symptomatology is dependent upon stage of disease. Patients may be diagnosed early secondary to PSA screening or have bone pain, weight loss, and fatigue associated with metastasis. Obstructive symptoms occur due to tumor growth locally and urinary retention is not uncommon.
- Diagnosis made on biopsy, primarily TRUS biopsy. PSA screening appropriate for:

  – All men 55–69 years old. 40–54 years old if high risk. Annual or every 2 years is appropriate.

- *Cystoscopic appearance*: The prostatic urethra will likely appear normal or with obstructing lobes with lower stage disease. More advanced stage disease may have an evident dysplastic appearance of the prostatic urethra.
- Treatment: Prostate cancer treatment is dependent upon the Gleason grade and the stage of the tumor.

Additional References for Consideration
- About Prostate Cancer American cancer society website.
- USCS Data Visualizations—CDC Statistics on Prostate Cancer.
- Campbell-Walsh-Wein Urology by Alan W. Partin MD, PhD, Roger R. Dmochowski D, MMHC, FACS, Louis R. Kavoussi MD, MBA, and Craig A. Peters M.
- Penn Clinical Manual of Urology by Philip M. Hanno MD, MPH, Thomas J. Guzzo MD, MPH, S. Bruce Malkowicz MD, and Alan J. Wein MD, FACS, PhD.

References

1. Geavlete P, Multescu R, Dragutescu M, Georgescu D, Geavlete B. Endoscopic treatment of urethral tumors. In: Geavlete P, editor. Endoscopic diagnosis and treatment in urethral pathology. London: Elsevier; 2021. p. 129–49.
2. Gillitzer R, Hampel C, Hadaschik B, Thuroff J. Single-institution experience with primary rumors of the male urethra. Br J Urol Int. 2008:964–8.
3. Anderson C, McKierman J. Tumors of the urethra. In: Partin A, Dmochowski R, Kavoussi L, Peters C, editors. Campbell-Walsh-Wein urology. Philadelphia: Elsevier; 2021. p. 1776–89.
4. Barocas DA, Boorjian SA, Alvarez RD, et al. Microhematuria: AUA/SUFU guideline. J Urol. 2020;204:778–86. Retrieved from American Urologic Association
5. Thyavihally Y, Tongaonkar H, Srivastava S, Raibhattanavar S. Clinical outcome of 36 male patients with primary urethral carcinoma: a single center experience. Int J Urol. 2006:716–20.
6. Guzzo T, Malkowicz B, Vaughn D, Wein A. Adult genitourinary cancer: prostate and bladder. In: Hanno P, Guzzo T, Malkowicz BW, editors. Penn clinical manual of urology. Philadelphia: Elsevier Inc; 2014. p. 505–8.
7. Centers for Disease Control and Prevention. (2021, June 8). *Prostate Cancer Statistics*. Retrieved from CDC https://www.cdc.gov/cancer/prostate/statistics/index.htm
8. American Urological Association. (2021). *Prostate Cancer Guidelines*. Retrieved from AUANET: https://www.auanet.org/guidelines/oncology-guidelines/prostate-cancer

Chapter 5
Benign Bladder Pathology

5.1 Acute Cystitis

5.1.1 Pathophysiology

Inflammation of the bladder can be secondary to infection, autoimmune disease, or injury. The most common cause of cystitis is infection, primarily due to bacteria. The most common bacterial organisms that cause genitourinary infections are the following: *E. coli* (85% of community-acquired infections and up to 50% of nosocomial infections), Proteus species, Klebsiella species, *Enterococcus faecalis*, and *Staphylococcus saprophyticus* [1].

In females, bacteria are aided access into the bladder by the short anatomical length of the urethra as well as the proximity to the vagina and rectum. This is one of the reasons why cystitis is much more common in females than in men. Cystitis in men is characterized as a complicated urinary tract infection warranting treatment. Not all female infections are complicated and thus not all female UTIs require treatment. Complicated urinary tract infections are those that include the following criteria: men, febrile infections, suspected urinary obstruction (can be due to tumor, calculi, stricture, etc.), immunocompromised state, atypical organisms, recurrent multidrug resistant organisms, infections post instrumentation, infections post genitourinary surgery, and lastly those with impaired renal function [2].

5.1.2 Clinical Presentation

Patients who are suffering from cystitis tend to have characteristic urinary symptoms. Symptoms specific to the urinary tract include the following: burning with urination/dysuria, urinary frequency, urinary urgency, sensation of incomplete

B. C. Tenny, M. O'Neill, *Diagnostic Cystoscopy*, https://doi.org/10.1007/978-3-031-10668-2_5

Table 5.1 The above table incorporates data adapted from (Ramakrishnan & Scheid, 2005)

	Sensitivity	Specificity
Bacteriuria	40–70%	85–95%
Pyuria	95%	71%
Dipstick nitrite +	45–60%	>85–98%
Dipstick leukocyte esterase +	48–86% *With nitrite + raises sensitivity to 68–88%	17–93%
>100,000 CFU on culture	Approx. 50%	>90%
>1000 CFU on culture	70–90% *Lowering cutoff for DX of UTI increases accuracy of test/more likely to detect an infection. However, risks false positives	High with symptoms

emptying, pain to the suprapubic region or flank, and hematuria. Symptoms in of themselves are not perfect in differentiating upper and lower tract involvement. Fevers, chills, and flank pain can indicate pyelonephritis; however, this triad has also been documented in isolated bladder infections as well. Furthermore, urine aspirate from the renal pelvis during cystitis has also been documented to yield positive urine cultures [3].

Diagnosis of a UTI can often be made based upon history alone of the above-mentioned symptoms. The clinician should consider an extra-vesicle etiology in patients that report vaginal irritation or vaginal discharge. Symptoms from cystitis are also typically more pronounced than those caused by urethritis. Urethritis can also cause burning with urination/dysuria, etc.

Diagnostic tests that assist in narrowing the differential diagnosis include a urinalysis and urine culture/gram stain. A urinalysis, "UA," includes the microscopic, macroscopic, and chemical evaluation of the patient's urine. Urine is examined for color/clarity, smell, trace minerals, presence of protein, identification of cells and microorganisms, and byproducts of cellular metabolism. The presence of WBCs (labeled "pyuria"), bacteria, leukocyte esterase, and nitrites should warrant suspicion of a urinary tract infection (see Table 5.1). The sensitivity and specificity of the UA in regard to infection are seen below:

5.1.3   Cystoscopic Image(s)

5.1.4   Suggested Treatments

Empirical treatment for a urinary tract infection is appropriate and does not necessarily warrant a urine culture for diagnosis. Duration of antimicrobial therapy is tailored towards the suspected organism and the chosen antibiotic.

Antibiotics:

Nitrofurantoin 100 mg PO BID for 5 days
Trimethoprim- sulfamethoxazole 800 mg/160 mg PO BID for three to 5 days
Cephalexin/cephalosporins 250 mg PO QID for three to 5 days
Ciprofloxacin/fluoroquinolones 500 mg PO BID for 3 days
Fosfomycin, single 3 gm IM single dose

Summary Key Points

- The most common bacterial organisms that cause genitourinary infections are the following: *E. coli* (85% of community-acquired and up to 50% of nosocomial infections), Proteus species, Klebsiella species, *Enterococcus faecalis*, and *Staphylococcus saprophyticus*.
- Symptoms specific to the urinary tract include the following: burning with urination/dysuria, urinary frequency, urinary urgency, sensation of incomplete emptying, pain to the suprapubic region or flank, and hematuria.
- Diagnosis: Urine analysis and urine culture.
- Cystoscopic appearance: Cystoscopy will likely demonstrate all or some of the following findings: turbid urine, hyperemia of bladder/confluence of vessels, mucosal edema, petechiae or hemorrhagic changes (see Figs. 5.1 and 5.2).
- Empirical treatment for a urinary tract infection is appropriate and does not necessarily warrant a urine culture for diagnosis.

Additional References for Consideration

- Penn Clinical Manual of Urology by Philip M. Hanno MD, MPH, Thomas J. Guzzo MD, MPH, S. Bruce Malkowicz MD and Alan J. Wein MD, FACS, PhD.
- Textbook of Family Medicine by Robert E. Rakel MD and David P. Rakel MD.

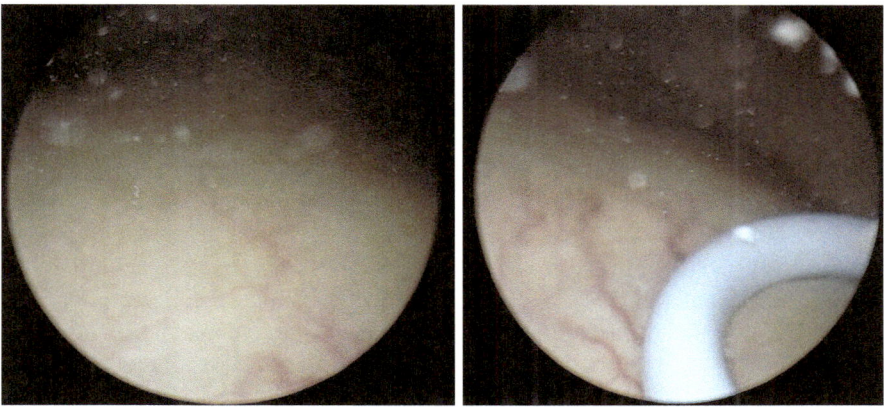

Fig. 5.1 Purulent urine in setting of a urinary tract infection. Left sided DJ stent was placed due to infected obstructing ureteral stone

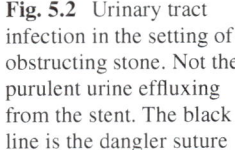

Fig. 5.2 Urinary tract infection in the setting of obstructing stone. Not the purulent urine effluxing from the stent. The black line is the dangler suture

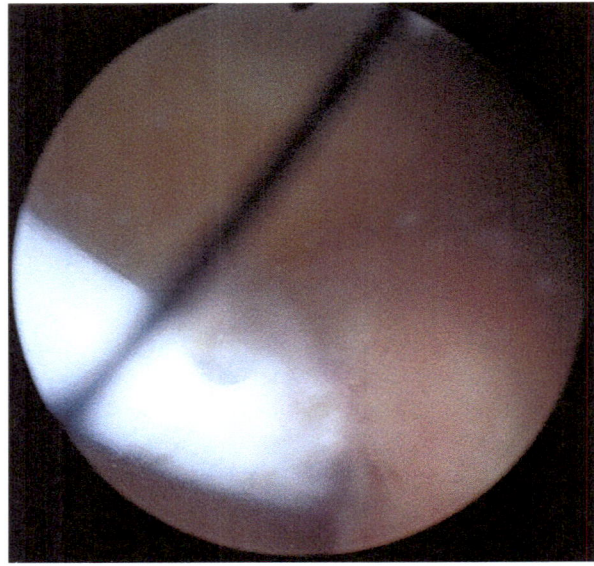

5.2   Inflammatory Tumors/Polyps

5.2.1   Pathophysiology

Benign bladder tumors or polyps occur due to inflammation. Polyps can arise in acute or chronic inflammation and are characterized by gross and histologic appearance. Examples include urothelial papilloma, inverted papilloma, nephrogenic adenoma, cystitis cystica/glandularis, xanthoma, leiomyoma, hemangioma, and neurofibroma.

Urothelial papilloma is a benign proliferative growth of epithelial cells/stalks that are encased in normal appearing urothelium causing a protrusion into the bladder's lumen. These lesions are benign without risk of malignant proliferation but share a fibroblast growth factor mutation with malignant bladder tumors (Montironi & Lopez-Beltran, 2005) (Kates & Bivalacqua, 2021).

Inverted papillomas are subcategorized, within the urothelial papilloma, once microscopy examination has identified an inverted histologic architecture versus the exophytic structure expected in polyp lesions (there is an endophytic structure with the epithelial cells invaginating into the lamina propria) (citation needed). Cystoscopy usually identifies inverted papillomas as a solitary sessile lesion, <3 cm, or with a short stalk occurring predominantly along the bladder trigone. Reoccurrence rate for inverted papillomas is <1% [4–6, 14].

Cystitis cystica is a benign pathology, which is cystoscopically characterized as a pearly white translucent cyst along the urothelium of the bladder (see Fig. 5.3). These lesions are typically found incidentally and are associated with infection/inflammation. Cystitis glandularis is a similar inflammatory process, involving

Fig. 5.3 Pictured above are cystic inflammatory lesions secondary to inflammation, usually infection, termed cystitis cystica

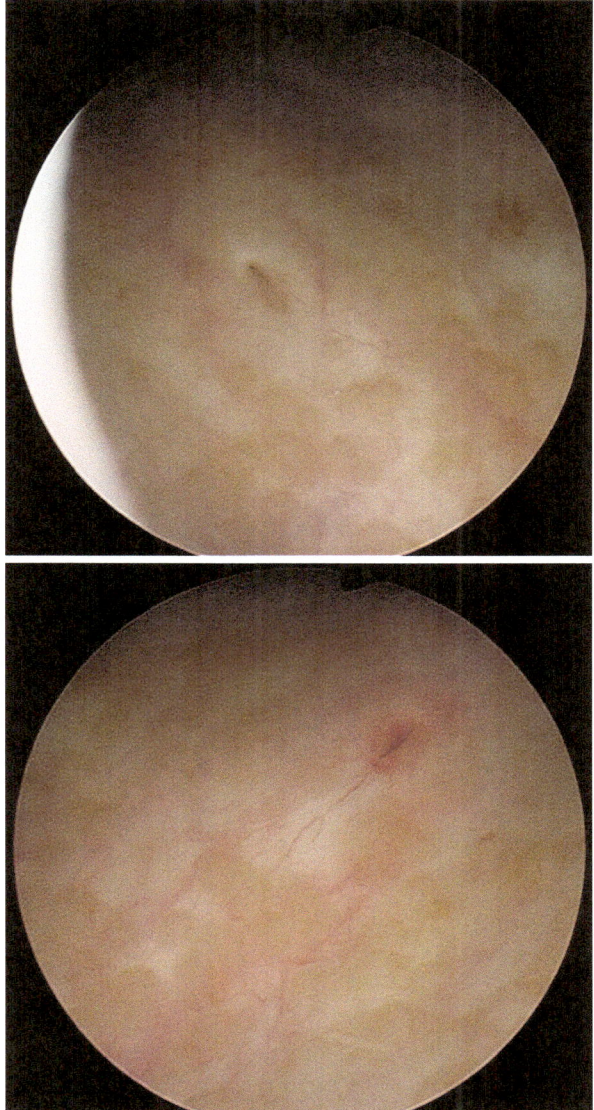

cystic proliferation of the urothelium. This lesion however is characterized by luminal cuboidal or columnar shaped epithelial cells (glandular cells) forming cysts, rather than normal cystic structure. Cystitis glandularis has a very small possible risk for adenocarcinoma formation if it is found to be the intestinal type with goblet cells [4–6, 14]. This association, however, is reported to be controversial.

Nephrogenic adenoma is a rare bladder tumor associated with chronic inflammation. These lesions also arise from the epithelial lining of the bladder but appear as immature renal tubules on microscopy. This is thought to be secondary to damage to the epithelial lining with subsequent seeding from displaced renal tubular cells. They are thus commonly associated with genitourinary surgery (including renal transplantation), intravesical chemotherapy use, catheters, or chronic infections [4]. Cystoscopically these lesions may be difficult to exclude from malignant tumors and biopsy is warranted (see Figs. 5.4 and 5.5).

Fig. 5.4 Pictured here is a benign bladder dome lesion. Histological examination demonstrated a congested lesion with coarse papillae largely denuded of epithelium, distorted epithelium. These features are suggestive of a nephrogenic adenoma. Recommendation is for repeat cystoscopic examination at an appropriate clinical interval

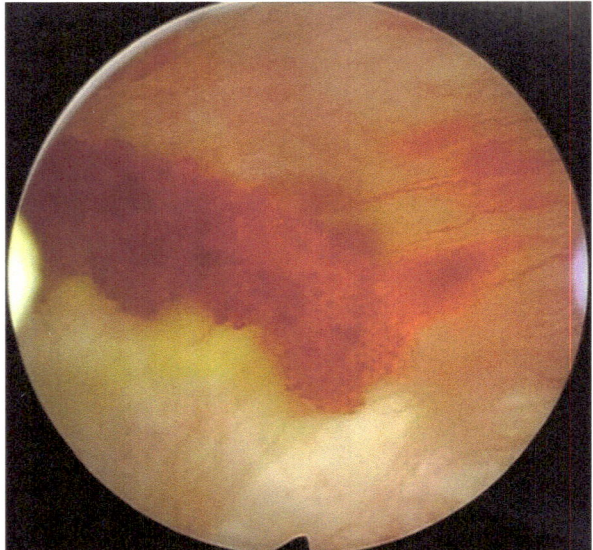

Fig. 5.5 On the posterior right bladder wall there was noted a erythematous, ulcerative lesion with sloughed mucosa. Histologic examination demonstrated ulcer with nephrogenic adenoma

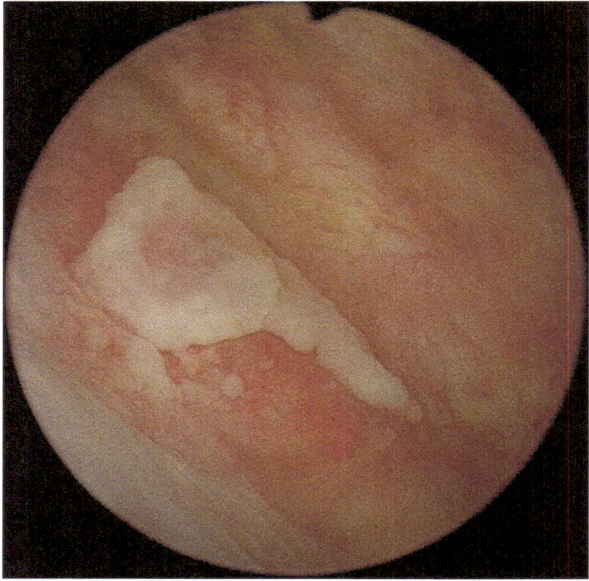

Urinary bladder xanthoma is a rare bladder lesion. It is associated with metabolic disorders that cause lipid accumulation within macrophages due to inflammation. Its appearance is that of a yellow plaque or papillary sessile lesion with ill-defined borders.

Leiomyoma of the bladder is the most common mesenchymal tumor found, although all bladder mesenchymal tumors are rare phenomena. The total incidence of mesenchymal tumors is approximately 0.5% of all bladder tumors [7]. Leiomyomas are typically found incidentally. Large tumors can manifest with lower urinary tract symptoms. Microscopically these tumors appear as a non-infiltrative smooth muscle cell lacking mitotic activity, cellular atypia, and necrosis. As a mesenchymal tumor they arise within the submucosa, the connective tissue, but can grow to the point of having an endophytic or exophytic papillary lesion. It is important to not confuse leiomyomas with leiomyosarcoma, which is malignant.

Hemangioma of the bladder typically manifests in children but can occur at any age. They have a male predilection of approx. 4:1. Painless gross hematuria is the most common symptom. These tumors can occur as isolated entities or associated with syndromes such as Sturge-Weber syndrome (congenital "port wine stain" on the forehead and brow). Diagnosis is made by biopsy; the clinician should be careful and monitor for gross hematuria post tissue retrieval [8].

Neurofibroma is a very rare nerve plexus tumor of the bladder. It can be associated with inheritable disorders, such as neurofibromatosis type 1. The bladder is the most common affected genitourinary organ if involved. The tumors typically arise along the bladder trigone, as this is the site of primary bladder nerve innervation. The tumors can grow within the bladder wall or be seen within the vesicle lumen. Neurofibromas can be localized, diffuse, or plexiform. [9].

5.2.2   Clinical Presentation

Benign tumors can manifest in similar fashion to malignant tumors of the bladder (see Fig. 5.6). There can be hematuria (either microscopic or gross), there can be lower urinary tract symptoms such as dysuria, incomplete emptying, and urinary frequency. Benign tumors that are not significantly large may be completely asymptomatic as well. Some tumors that are primarily benign have a rare incidence of malignant progression and removal with subsequent surveillance cystoscopy may be warranted.

Fig. 5.6 Cystoscopy for a
bladder mass revealed a
bladder wall granuloma
that corresponded to the
proximal area of the
extraperitoneal bladder
injury the patient had
months prior. Histology
following resection
confirmed granulation like
tissue with focal foreign
body giant cell reaction;
benign bladder tissue

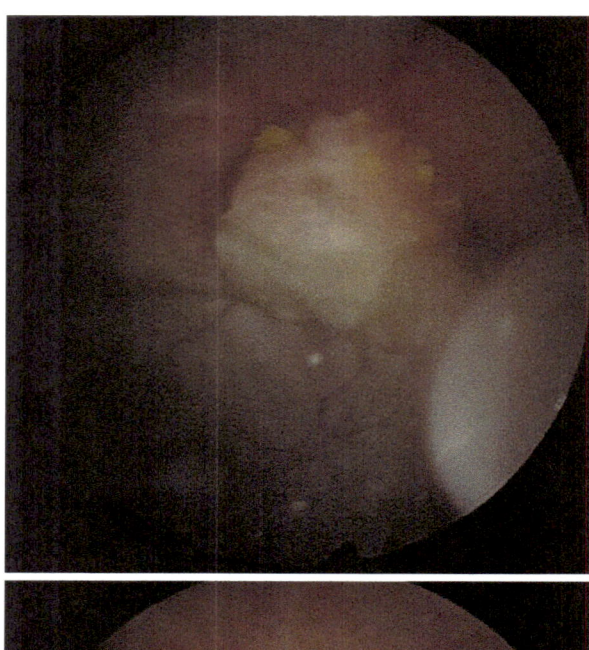

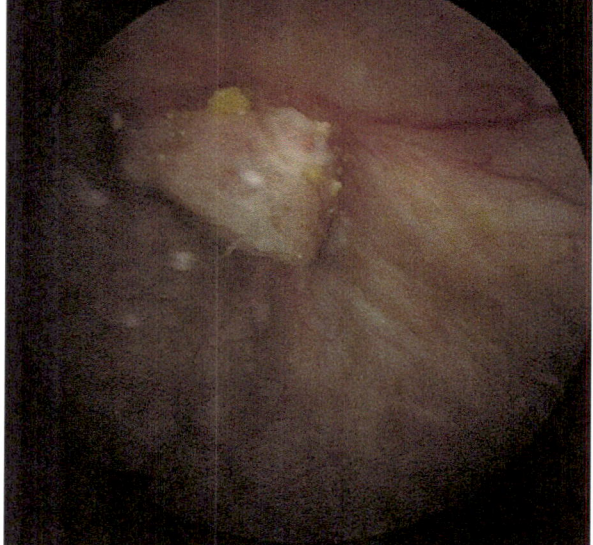

5.2.3 Cystoscopic Image(s)

5.2.4 Suggested Treatments

If found incidentally and known to be a benign lesion without concern for malignancy, no treatment may be appropriate. Interventions, although performed frequently, are not without possible risks of injury, such as bladder perforation or

significant hematuria. Patient's that are symptomatic should be treated with tumor resection as this may improve the patient's quality of life.

Summary Key Points

- Benign bladder tumors arise in acute or chronic inflammation and are characterized by gross and histologic appearance.

    - Urothelial papilloma is a benign proliferative growth of epithelial cells/stalks that are encased in normal appearing urothelium causing a protrusion into the bladder's lumen.
    - Inverted papillomas are a urothelial papilloma with inverted histologic architecture. Cystoscopy usually identifies these as a solitary sessile lesion, <3 cm, or with a short stalk occurring predominantly along the bladder trigone.
    - Nephrogenic Adenomas are rare. Commonly associated with renal transplantation (thought to be due to damage and seeding of renal epithelial cells), intravesical chemotherapy use, catheters, and chronic infections. Difficult to exclude from malignant appearing lesions.
    - Cystitis cystica, characterized as superficial pearly white translucent cysts. Found with active inflammation or infection.

        Cystitis glandularis, similar to cystitis cystica, but characterized by luminal cuboidal or columnar shaped epithelial cells forming cysts versus normal cystic structure. With glandularis, controversial association (very rare) risk of adenocarcinoma formation.

    - Xanthoma rare. Associated with metabolic disorders/lipid accumulation in macrophages. Yellow plaque or yellow papillary sessile lesion with ill-defined borders.
    - Leiomyoma, exceedingly rare (<0.5% of all bladder tumors). Do NOT confuse with leiomyo*sarcoma* which is malignant.
    - Hemangioma, manifest in children primarily. Male predominance (4:1). Associated with painless gross hematuria. Can be associated with syndromes: Sturge-Weber syndrome.
    - Neurofibroma, very rare nerve plexus tumor of the bladder. Can be associated with inheritable disorders.

- If found incidentally and *known* to be a benign lesion without concern for malignancy, no treatment may be appropriate. Otherwise, resection for histological assessment and fulguration is appropriate.

Additional References for Consideration

- Urothelial papilloma—American Urological Association (auanet.org)
- Inverted papilloma—American Urological Association (auanet.org)
- Inverted urothelial papilloma—StatPearls—NCBI Bookshelf (nih.gov)
- Nephrogenic adenoma—American Urological Association (auanet.org)
- Cystitis glandularis—American Urological Association (auanet.org)
- Xanthoma of the urinary bladder—PubMed (nih.gov)
- Xanthoma of the urinary bladder—A rare entity—PubMed (nih.gov)

5.3   Hemorrhagic Cystitis

5.3.1   *Pathophysiology*

Hemorrhagic cystitis is defined by diffuse bladder inflammation with associated hematuria. Hematuria should be visible on gross exam with the severity of inflammation ranging from a transient process to one requiring surgical intervention (see Figs. 5.7 and 5.8). Causes include infection from microorganisms or viruses, trauma,

Fig. 5.7 Cystoscopy demonstrated radiation cystitis involvement of the trigone and posterior bladder wall (the bladder dome and lateral walls were noted to be spared). There was successful treatment/hemostasis with the cautery Bugbee probe

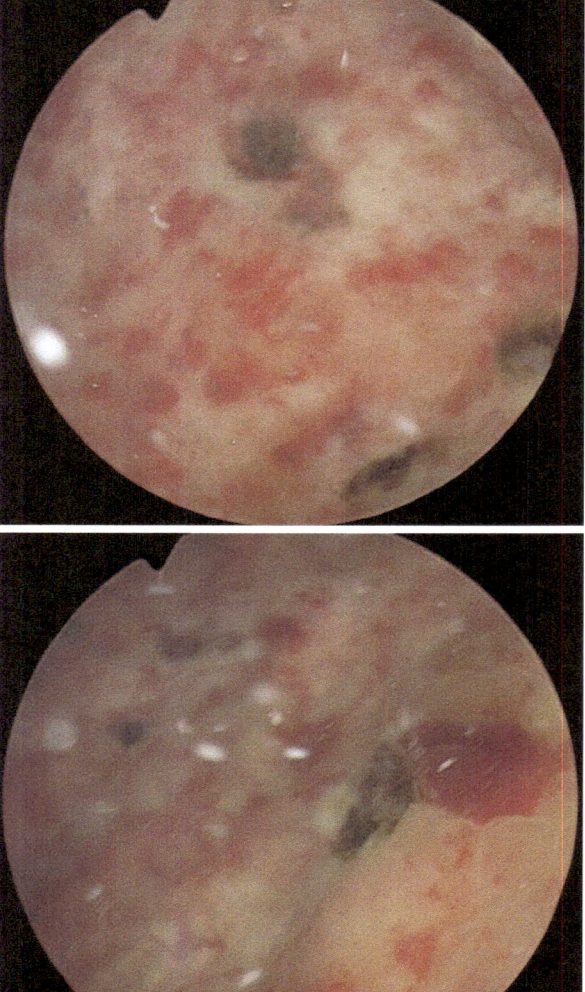

Fig. 5.8 Bullous mucosal edema with an adherent clot. Diagnosis was hemorrhagic cystitis and required clot evacuation as well as fulguration for treatment

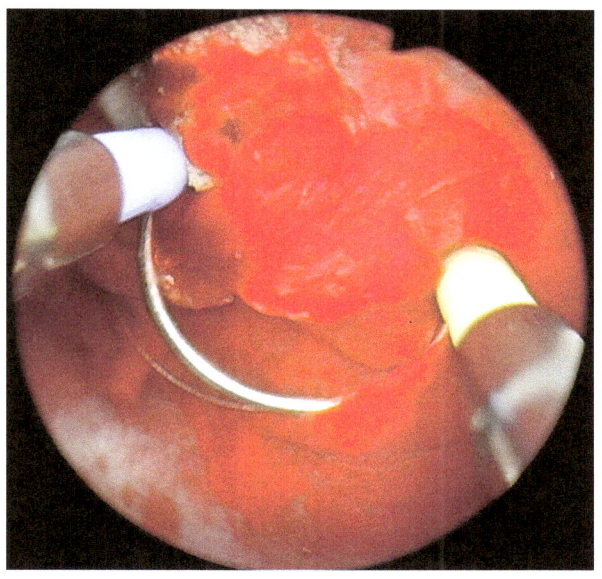

malignancy, chemical exposure, prior irradiation, or manifestation of systemic disease. One commonly implicated virus in children or immunocompromised adults is the BK virus.

Chemicals that have been implicated include chemotherapy, such as cyclophosphamide and ifosfamide, ether, bleomycin, and aniline dye. The risk of hemorrhagic cystitis following cyclophosphamide and ifosfamide is so great that literature has shown that up to 40% of patients who received this form of chemotherapy may have this complication; there is, however, a dose-dependent relationship [10] (Brade, Herdrich, & Varini, 1985).

Preventative measures while undergoing chemotherapy include the administration of 2-mercaptoethan sulfonate (Mesna), which binds to acrolein in the urologic tract leaving it inactive, and hyperhydration with forced diuresis with/without Foley catheter placement. These measures are not foolproof and a reported 10–40% of patients will still develop hemorrhagic cystitis [11].

Radiation causes hemorrhagic cystitis by direct damage to the vascular and mucosal endothelium. Radiation cystitis on cystoscopy will be less diffuse and more localized to the wall of the bladder where the radiation had passed through it.

5.3.2   Clinical Manifestations

Again, patients will experience gross hematuria that will either be transient and resolve spontaneously or require surgery with fulguration. Patients may experience hematuria 48 hrs following administration of chemotherapy or several years following. Those who have had prior radiation treatment to present several months to years following therapy [12].

Diagnosis is made based upon the typical clinical presentation, and a thorough history should be performed to narrow down the etiology. If infection is present, the patient should be treated appropriately. Viral infections typically spontaneously resolve; however, they can be severe enough to warrant instrumentation. Antivirals have had documented success in treating the BK virus and adenovirus type 11 etiology.

5.3.3 Cystoscopic Image(s)

5.3.4 Suggested Treatments

The initial management of patients with hematuria is ensuring adequate bladder drainage. Urinary obstruction can precipitate renal injury and thus hinder other necessary medical treatment while the kidneys are under stress. Alleviating bladder outlet obstruction can be done by passage of a large bore Foley catheter, >22 French foley; however, it needs to be done again only if the hematuria is severe with evident clots.

Hematuria can be severe enough to cause anemia, and serial complete blood counts should be done to ensure that this does not occur. Other laboratory workup would include urinalysis, urine culture, and possible viral panel to ascertain etiology if the history intake is not significant. If infection is present, treat cause. Again, viral infections are typically transient but the usage of antivirals such as Leflunomide has had reported success [13].

The determination for surgery is usually made after continuous bladder irrigation fails to allow for bladder healing/hematuria resolution. Diluting the urine and ensuring no clot retention by continuous irrigation can allow for the mucosal lining of the bladder to heal. If the patient requires repeat bedside manual irrigation or has required multiple transfusions, the decision to proceed to surgery should not be delayed. Cystoscopy with clot evacuation and fulguration may need to be repeated more than once in severe settings.

Adjunct measures typically performed prior to or after surgery, include intravesical instillation of agents that decrease fibrinolysis (Aminocaproic acid) and astringents (alum and silver nitrate), hyperbaric oxygen, administration of intravesical formalin, selective iliac artery embolization, and possibly cystectomy with urinary diversion. The latter intervention is seldomly performed and usually in the setting of severe trauma that would warrant cystectomy anyway.

Summary Key Points
- Hemorrhagic cystitis is diffuse bladder inflammation with associated hematuria.

  - Causes include infection from microorganisms or viruses (ex: BK virus), trauma, malignancy, chemical exposure (ex: cyclophosphamide or aniline dyes), prior irradiation, or manifestation of systemic disease.

    Radiation etiology can result in Hematuria that presents years later after therapy.

- Patients will present with frank hematuria and/or clot retention. It is important to assess for the above risk factors, although conservative measures are unlikely to drastically defer between causes: large borer catheter, manual irrigation, and continuous bladder irrigation.
- *Cystoscopic appearance*: Hemorrhagic cystitis will appear as diffuse bladder inflammation/hemorrhagic changes coupled with impressive hematuria. Hematuria may wax and wane dependent upon intravesical clot presence. Radiation cystitis appears similar; however, the inflammation is localized to the wall where the radiation traveled through.
- Treatment is directed towards assisting bladder drainage and preventing severe anemia. Treating causes, such as abx for UTI and antivirals for BK virus infection, is appropriate as well. It is very common for patients needing to go to the OR for a clot evacuation.

Additional References for Consideration
- Campbell-Walsh-Wein Urology by Alan W. Partin MD, PhD, Roger R. Dmochowski D, MMHC, FACS, Louis R. Kavoussi MD, MBA, and Craig A. Peters M.
- Chemotherapy and radiation-related hemorrhagic cystitis in cancer patients—UpToDate.

5.4   Metaplasia of the Bladder/Flat Lesions

5.4.1   Pathophysiology

Metaplasia is defined as an abnormal change of mature adult cells of a tissue to another cell type (see Figs. 5.9 and 5.10). In the bladder this occurs on the transitional epithelial mucosal layer and typically at the site of the bladder trigone. Transitional epithelial cells can change into squamous epithelial cells or glandular epithelial cells (see Fig. 5.11). The former type is very common, affecting 40% of women and 5% of men; the change occurs from inflammation due to infection, trauma, or prior surgery (Ozbey, Aksoy, Polat, & al, 1993). This disorder is a benign process and requires no treatment.

Fig. 5.9 Mucosal metaplasia characterized by a white thickened patch of urothelium. Seen at 6 o'clock along the trigone ridge

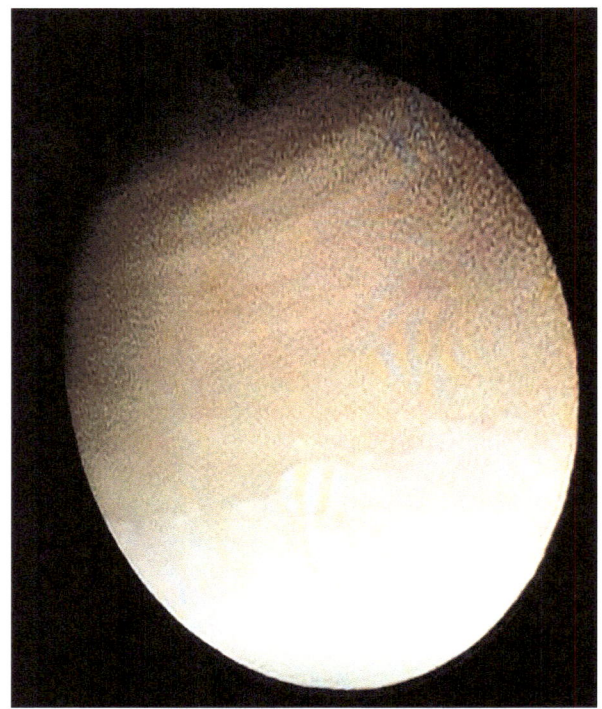

Fig. 5.10 Left ureteral orifice with mucosal metaplasia along the trigone and bladder neck, pictured at 6 o'clock

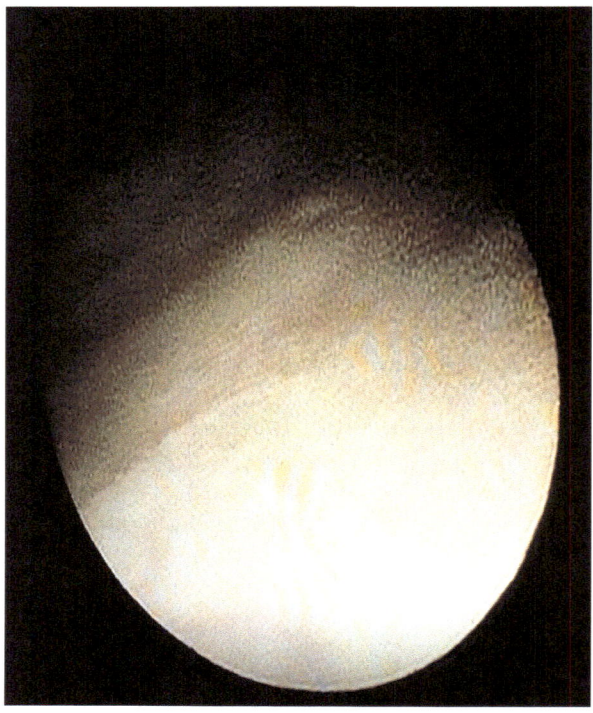

Fig. 5.11 Cystoscopy for microscopic hematuria. Noted small bladder neck polyps along the junction of the anterior wall. Resection and histologic examination revealed cystitis cystica with nonkeratinizing squamous metaplasia

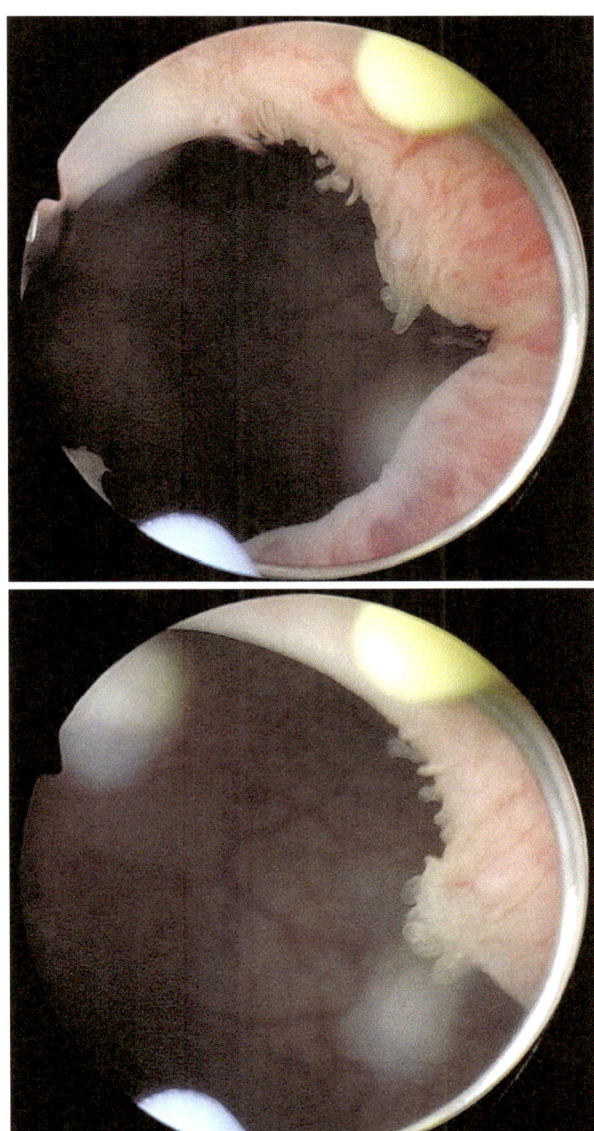

This inflammation can occur with leukoplakia, which are thickened white patches that may be floating or along the mucosal surface. The leukoplakia within in the bladder has not been shown to have malignant progression (Staack, Schlechte, Sachs, & al, 2006). Furthermore, squamous metaplasia can be sub-characterized by the presence of keratin (see Fig. 5.12). Nonkeratinizing squamous metaplasia as described above is considered a normal clinical finding resulting from inflammation. Disposition of keratin with metaplasia, however, is associated with subsequent squamous dysplasia, and there is suggestion as noting this as a precursor lesion for carcinoma [4–6, 14].

Fig. 5.12 Carpeted keratinizing squamous metaplasia, with an atypical blue hue. Said patient had resection/ biopsy of the above lesion given the variant color found with histologic examination confirming the benign process. Repeat cystoscopy 3 months post initial resection and fulguration demonstrated no residual nor reoccurrence of the lesion

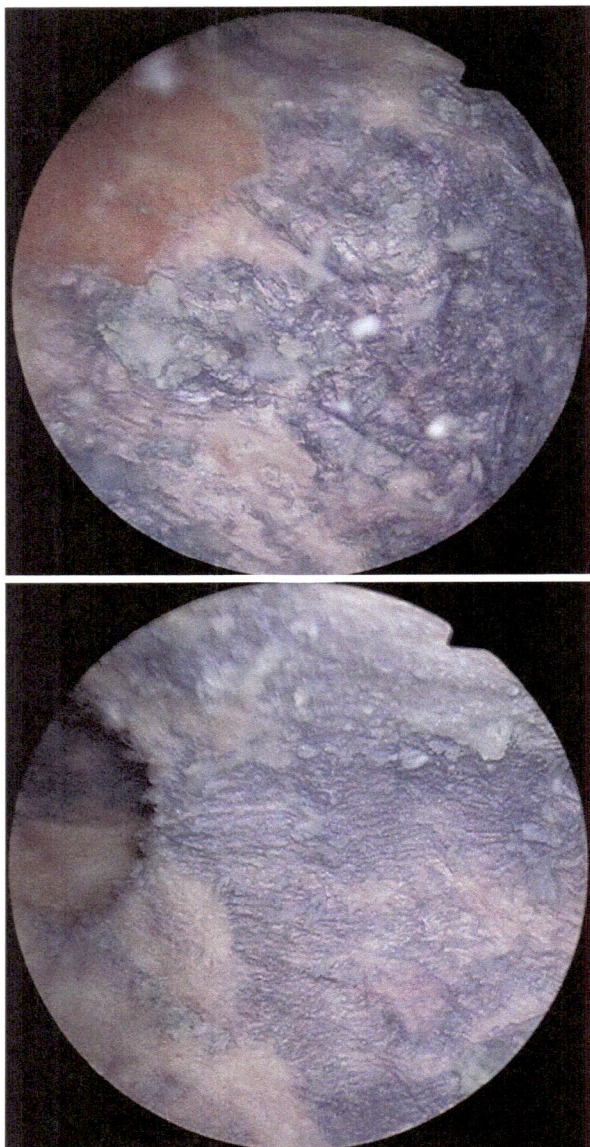

5.4.2   Clinical Presentation

Metaplasia is typically found incidentally. It is highly prevalent in women and is also found in men. Commonly associated features are a history of recurrent urinary tract infections, prior bladder surgery, or bladder trauma.

5.4.3 Cystoscopic Image(s)

Summary Key Points
- Metaplasia is an abnormal change in the transitional epithelial mucosal layer of the bladder to squamous epithelial or glandular epithelial cells.

    - Very common, approx. 40% of women and 5% of men. Occurs due to inflammation.
    - Can occur with leukoplakia (no malignant potential) or keratin disposition (is associated with dysplasia but questionable association to subsequent malignancy).

- Patients may be asymptomatic or present with irritative urologic symptoms. Diagnosis only confirmed on cystoscopy.
- *Cystoscopic appearance*: A white (predominantly) carpeted thickened plaque with mucosal desquamation. Primarily occurring at the base of the bladder along the trigone or near the bladder neck.
- No treatment necessary.

Suggested Treatments
At this current moment no treatment is recommended for metaplasia of the bladder.

Additional References for Consideration
- Squamous Metaplasia—American Urological Association (auanet.org).
- Campbell-Walsh-Wein Urology by Alan W. Partin MD, PhD, Roger R. Dmochowski D, MMHC, FACS, Louis R. Kavoussi MD, MBA, and Craig A. Peters M.

5.5 Interstitial Cystitis/Bladder Pain Syndrome

5.5.1 Pathophysiology

Interstitial cystitis or more commonly known as bladder pain syndrome (IC/BPS) is defined as "an unpleasant sensation (pain, pressure, discomfort) perceived to be related to the urinary bladder, associated with lower urinary tract symptoms of more than 6 weeks duration, in absence of infection or identifiable causes" (The Society for Urodynamics and Female Urology, 2012). Overactive bladder should be excluded while diagnosing IC/BPS; however, 14% of BPS patients have been found to have urodynamic overactivity. The definition is purposefully broad in order to include those who have overt inflammation and those with reported pain without any observable inflammatory markers [15].

Not a lot is known regarding pathophysiology of this disease process. A proposed, "leaky epithelium" secondary to mast cell activation, neurogenic inflammation, infection, and primary pelvic floor dysfunction have all been proposed as an etiology of initial and subsequent chronic bladder inflammation [16].

Histologically there is no pathognomonic criteria for IC/BPS. IC/BPS is thus a heterogenous syndrome characterized by the aforementioned definition [15]. There have been discoveries of an antiproliferative factor (APF), made by Dr. Susan Keay et al., that appears to impede the growth of cell culture from the bladder lining in IC/BPS patients. This APF has been found in the urine of IC/BPS bladders rather than the renal pelvis indicating that the bladder is likely the source of production. Subsequent studies have demonstrated that APF is associated with a decrease in heparin-binding EGF like growth factor and an increase in epidermoid growth factor and insulin like growth factor. The disturbance in these enzymes is postulated to prevent epithelial proliferation resulting in IC/BPS in patients who unfortunately experience some nidus of inflammation or injury [16].

5.5.2   Clinical Presentation

The essential condition of IC/BPS is discomfort associated with the bladder. The discomfort is characterized by worsening severity with reported bladder filling. The discomfort can be experienced as pain and/or pressure. This may result in urinary frequency and irritative voiding. Urine studies should be negative for infection, as the IC/BPS is a diagnosis of exclusion (definition states "in the absence of infection or identifiable causes"). Pain should be chronic rather than acute, with frequency of discomfort occurring at least episodically over 6 weeks [16].

Diagnostic studies are limited; however, rule in the diagnosis of IC/BPS but excluding other identifiable causes. The use of an intravesical potassium chloride solution has historically been performed; however, due to a low sensitivity and specificity it has fallen out of favor. The AUA does not recommend its use.

Drugs known to cause inflammation of the bladder, which may present similar to ICS/BPS, such as cyclophosphamide, aspirin, NSAIDs, allopurinol, and ketamine, should be excluded in the history intake. If the presence of hematuria is discovered, cystoscopy should be done to rule out bladder cancer; carcinoma in situ is known to cause similar symptoms.

Cystoscopy is performed to rule in the diagnosis by complete bladder examination while performing hydrodistension. Hydrodistension occurs with the instillation of 80-100 mm H20 pressure; this distention is also reported to alleviate the symptoms in patients with IC/BPS. When the bladder is stretched there may appear diffuse glomerulations (petechial bleeding points) or a localized circumscribed erythematous area of bleeding known as a Hunner lesion (HLs) (see Figs. 5.13 and 5.14). HLs is only present in approx. 10% of cases, and thus the symptomatology should primarily guide the diagnosis of the syndrome [17].

Fig. 5.13 Hunner's ulcer identified on cystoscopy. This Hunner's lesion has central desquamation of the mucosal layer; however, they can also appear as a circumscribed red lesion

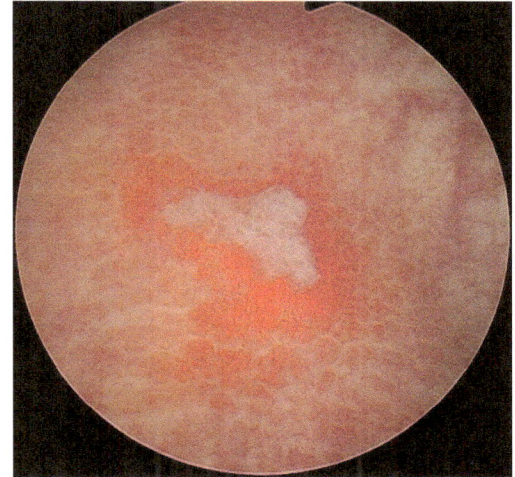

Fig. 5.14 Bladder glomerulations, or petechial hemorrhages, seen on the bladder wall of a patient undergoing hydrodistension to treat interstitial cystitis

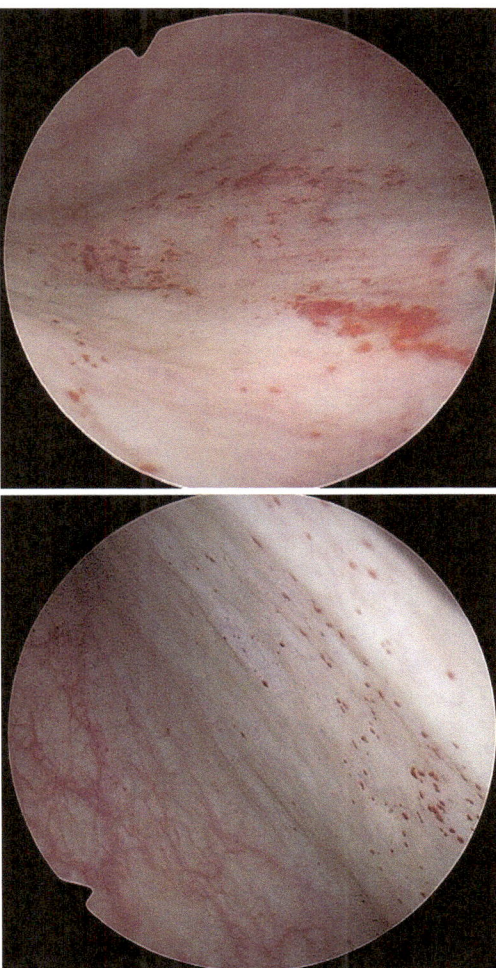

5.5.3   Cystoscopic Image(s)

5.5.4   Suggested Treatments

After diagnosis the decision is then made on whether to proceed with treatment. If the patient has not been on any empiric course of antibiotics it would be prudent to consider a standard course. Symptoms that are mild, that reportedly do not interfere with patient's quality of life (for example, minimal or scant nocturia, or pressure causing urinary frequency q3-4hrs), may not significantly improve with medicine. Furthermore, the medications recommended for administration can have intolerable side effects (tricyclic antidepressants).

Timed voiding and fluid intake modification can help patients with mild disease. Avoiding bladder irritants, such as caffeine, alcohol, and acidic beverages, may additionally help. Pelvic floor rehabilitation with myofascial trigger point release and intravaginal Thiele massage can reduce symptomatology with little side effects [18].

Many patients, however, require pharmacological therapy. Oral medication therapy includes amitriptyline, pentosan polysulfate sodium, and hydroxyzine. These medicines can be used concomitantly to reduce side effects from higher individual doses.

Patients with refractory or breakthrough symptoms will undergo cystoscopy, treatment/resection, and fulguration of Hunner lesions if present, along with instillation of intravesical medicine aimed at reducing inflammation and providing a protective covering of the exposed bladder epithelial layer. Intradetrusor botulinum toxin can be combined and performed along with hydrodistension; however, the patient must be willing and able to perform self-catheterization as there is a risk of urinary retention. The last-ditch effort is cystectomy with urinary diversion. This measure is reserved for severe cases of IC/BPS, and patients typically have an end-stage bladder (low bladder compliance; <200 cc) [15].

Summary Key Points
- IC/BPS is any unpleasant sensation, including pain, pressure, and discomfort related to the bladder lasting longer than 6 weeks in duration, in the absence of infection or other identifiable causes.

  - Important to exclude OAB; however, 14% of BPS patients have been found to have urodynamic overactivity.
  - Historically thought to be secondary to a "leaky epithelium" caused by inflammation with associated pelvic floor dysfunction. Discovery of the antiproliferative factor has demonstrated a biologic pathology that prevents epithelial proliferation.

- Chief complaint is bladder pain, pressure, or discomfort that progresses with bladder filling. This can then result in urinary frequency and irritative voiding. The discomfort should be chronic occurring at least episodically over 6 weeks.
- Diagnostics: Urine analysis and culture should be utilized to exclude active UTI. Cystoscopy is performed to rule in the diagnosis.
- *Cystoscopic appearance*: With hydrodistension there may appear diffuse glomerulations (petechial bleeding points) or a localized circumscribed erythematous area of bleeding known as a Hunner lesion (HLs). HLs are only present in 10%.
- Treatment can be performed on diagnosis with hydrodistension. Conservative therapy is appropriate for mild disease; such as tricyclic antidepressants, timed voiding, fluid intake modification, and avoiding of irritants. Refractory or breakthrough disease will benefit from cystoscopy hydrodistension, fulguration of any HLs, intradetrusor botulinum infections, and for last resort cystectomy with urinary diversion.

Additional References for Consideration
- Campbell-Walsh-Wein Urology by Alan W. Partin MD, PhD, Roger R. Dmochowski D, MMHC, FACS, Louis R. Kavoussi MD, MBA, and Craig A. Peters M.
- Penn Clinical Manual of Urology by Philip M. Hanno MD, MPH, Thomas J. Guzzo MD, MPH, S. Bruce Malkowicz MD and Alan J. Wein MD, FACS, PhD.

5.6   Bladder Trabeculations

5.6.1   Pathophysiology

Trabeculae are defined as cords or bands of connective tissue. These cords have a physiologic process with muscle tissue, similar to tendons, allowing for adequate contraction of the involved organ. In the heart they allow for a sufficient ejection fraction to ensure a low residual of blood remains in the ventricles. In the bladder, however, they are nearly always seen with obstruction. Normally the bladder's muscle is free of significant trabeculae forming a smooth hollow organ, but in clinical scenarios with chronic obstruction they result to assist with detrusor muscle contraction (see Fig. 5.15). This adaptive change is associated with hypertrophied smooth muscle of the bladder initially followed by excessive collagen deposition [19].

Fig. 5.15 Trabeculations of the bladder, seen as a non-smooth contour, on cystogram through a suprapubic catheter. Recent scholarly attempts at grading bladder trabeculations on cystogram have been made. A proposed grading system 0–2: 0) meaning smooth walled bladder, (1) bladder demonstrates shallow cellules/crevices or small diverticula, and (2) bladder wall demonstrating deep cellules or diverticula. Per the grading system proposed by Shelby and et al., this above cystogram would grade as a grade 2 (Shelby, Hidas, Chunag, & et al. 2020)

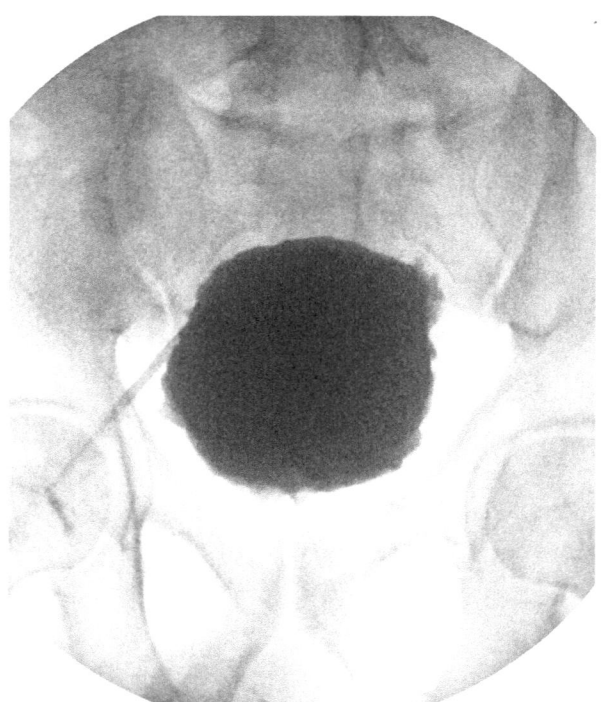

5.6.2   Clinical Presentation

Severe trabeculation is associated with an elevated residual urine/incomplete emptying (see Figs. 5.16 and 5.17). Patients will likely endorse obstructive lower urinary tract symptoms such as, needing to empty after having just gone to the bathroom, dribbling, and straining with urination. Bladder trabeculae are primarily identified on cystoscopy; however, they can be seen on cystograms.

5.6.3   Cystoscopic Image(s)

5.6.4   Suggested Treatments

Treatments for bladder trabeculations are aimed at the etiology for the bladder muscle hypertrophy. This can include either outlet procedures such as direct visualization internal urethrotomy, urethroplasty, and transurethral resection of the prostate.

Summary Key Points
- Bladder trabeculae are cords or bands of connective tissue that develop under chronically high outlet pressures requiring hypertrophy and increased contractility of the bladder.

Fig. 5.16 Female bladder seen with trabeculations on the posterior left lateral wall indicating possible outlet resistance

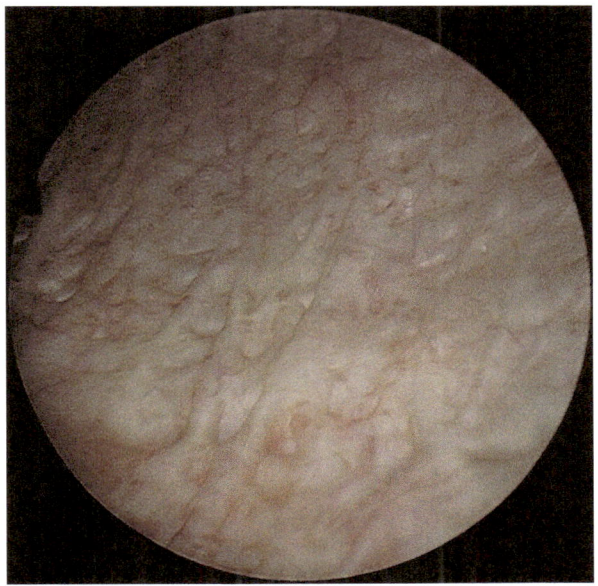

- Patients will likely endorse obstructive lower urinary tract symptoms. Severe trabeculations are associated with elevated residual urine levels/incomplete emptying.
- Easily diagnosed on cystoscopy and cystograms. There have been endeavors to grade bladder trabeculation; however, this has not yet been widely adopted.

  – A proposed grading system 0–2: 0) smooth walled bladder, (1) shallow cellules/crevices or small diverticula, and (2) bladder wall demonstrating deep cellules or diverticula.

- *Cystoscopic appearance*: The urothelium will depict a net like band structure underneath mucosa. Larger bands or cords will be evident with more severe trabeculations. This will result in either shallow or deep cellules.
- Treatment is aimed at fixing the cause of the high pressure in the bladder; bladder outlet obstruction. It is important to assess that the bladder still functions if the patient has severe trabeculations prior to intervention.

Additional References for Consideration Penn Clinical Manual of Urology by Philip M. Hanno MD, MPH, Thomas J. Guzzo MD, MPH, S. Bruce Malkowicz MD and Alan J. Wein MD, FACS, PhD.

- Campbell-Walsh-Wein Urology by Alan W. Partin MD, PhD, Roger R. Dmochowski D, MMHC, FACS, Louis R. Kavoussi MD, MBA, and Craig A. Peters M.

Fig. 5.17 Large bladder
trabeculations resulting in
formation of a deep cellule
in two separate patients

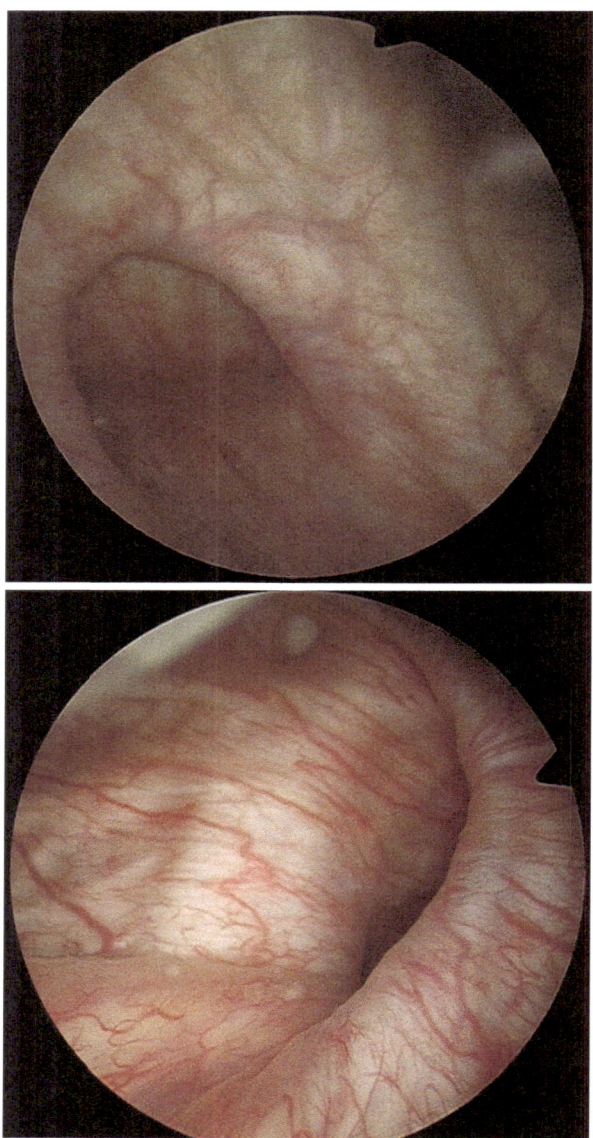

5.7   Bladder Diverticulum

5.7.1   Pathophysiology

As previously described a diverticulum is a protrusion of the most luminal/superfi-
cial layer through the smooth muscle layer, resulting in an extrinsic contained pouch
devoid of functional muscle layer (see Fig. 5.18). In the bladder, this pouch is

Fig. 5.18 Large bladder diverticulum with evident severe trabeculations secondary to long-standing outlet obstruction

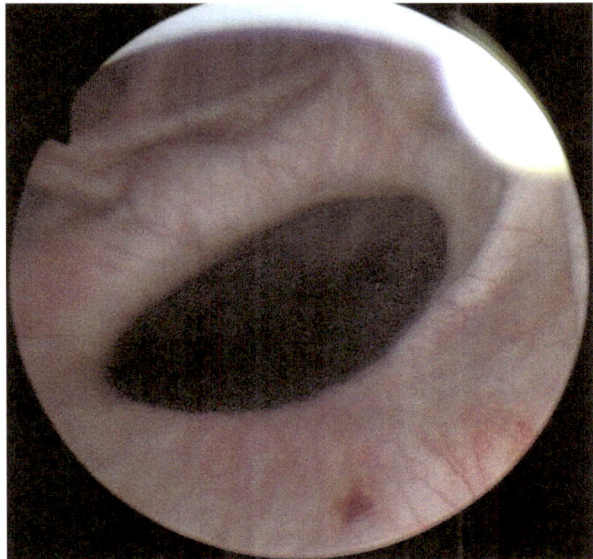

Fig. 5.19 Large bladder diverticulum along the left lateral wall

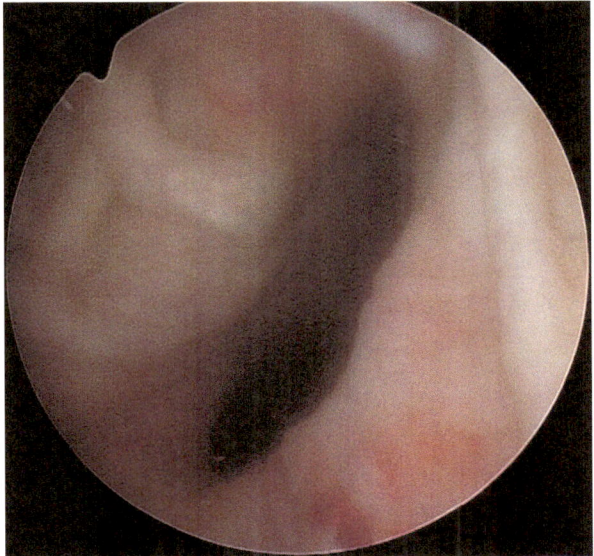

composed of two primary layers, the mucosa and underlying lamina propria tissue; but can additionally be contained within the final adventitial/fibrous capsule of the bladder (Shah & Richstone, 2021). Given that this area is primarily lacking in any smooth muscle, there may be scattered detrusor muscle fibers but there is no coordinated contraction, the pouch is functionally inert. This results in urinary stasis leading to stone formation and recurrent urinary tract infections (see Fig. 5.19).

In the adult patient, bladder diverticulum is primarily acquired resulting from long-standing outlet obstruction. There is a male predominance given benign prostatic hyperplasia causing the majority of bladder outlet obstruction.

5.7.2 Clinical Presentation

The majority of bladder diverticula are asymptomatic, only being discovered on radiographic imaging or cystoscopic examination. Symptoms that do occur result from the sequela of urinary stasis. Patients may have recurrent urinary tract infections despite adequate antibiotic treatment, they may present with a symptom of incomplete emptying and/or urinary frequency, foul smelling urine, and lastly symptoms suggestive of bladder calculi.

5.7.3 Cystoscopic Image(s)

5.7.4 Suggested Treatments

Management of patients with bladder diverticula include observation, endoscopic management, and surgical excision. Observation is appropriate for patients with minimal symptoms, no evidence of upper urinary tract injury, no evidence of malignancy, no diverticulum stones, and chronic relapsing urinary tract infection.

If a procedural intervention is warranted per the above problems, the clinician can consider either an endoscopic treatment or surgical excision. Endoscopic resection of the diverticular neck is preferable for patients who are too debilitated for primary surgery or those already undergoing therapy to treat the outlet obstruction.

Operative excision can be performed either open approach, laparoscopic, or robotically with or without concomitant outlet obstruction therapy (Shah & Richstone, 2021).

Summary Key Points
- A bladder diverticulum is a protrusion of the most luminal/superficial layer through the smooth muscle layer, resulting in a pouch devoid of any functional muscle layer.

  – Acquired diverticulum occurs due to long-standing outlet obstruction.

- Most patients are asymptomatic; however, there may be complaints of recurrent urinary tract infections, foul smelling urine, symptoms suggestive of bladder calculi, and of course obstructive lower urinary tract symptoms.

- Diagnosis can be made on either cystogram or cystoscopy.
- *Cystoscopic appearance:* On cystoscopy there will be an apparent large or small os leading to contained cavity or pouch within the bladder. There may or may not be associated trabeculations of the bladder.
- Treatments for the sequela of a bladder diverticula include observation, endoscopic management, and surgical excision. Observation is appropriate if minimal symptoms, no renal impairment, no malignancy, no diverticular stones, and no chronic relapsing urinary tract infection.

Additional References for Consideration
- Campbell-Walsh-Wein Urology by Alan W. Partin MD, PhD, Roger R. Dmochowski D, MMHC, FACS, Louis R. Kavoussi MD, MBA, and Craig A. Peters M

5.8 Bladder Fistula (Vesicovaginal and Vesicoenteric)

5.8.1 Pathophysiology

Fistulas are any extra-anatomic communication between two adjacent body structures. The most common site of urogenital fistula is between the bladder and the vagina, termed vesicovaginal fistula (VV fistula). Other fistulas' connections between the bladder are vesicoenteric (intestinal tract) (see Figs. 5.20 and 5.21) and less commonly vesico-uterine (uterus). Due to the low incidence of vesicouterine fistulas we will primarily discuss VV fistulas and vesicoenteric fistulas. Fistulous formation occurs due to localized tissue damage between two structures; the tissue damage can result from either iatrogenic injury such as following surgery or radiation, be a congenital anomaly (rare), occur due to prolonged childbirth (maternal injury), result from malignancy (responsible for 20% of all genitourinary enteric fistulas), or secondary to chronic inflammation [20].

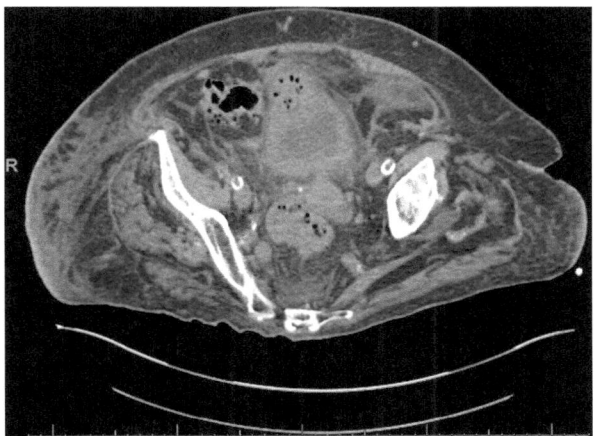

Fig. 5.20 CT scan of a patient with a confirmed bladder fistula. Seen here is a thickened/inflamed bowel loop adjacent to right anterior wall of the bladder. Air can be seen immediately extra-vesicle in the bladder's anterior plane

Fig. 5.21 Sagittal view of the same patient, picture above, with two findings confirming a fistula: 1. an adjacent inflamed/thickened bowel loop. 2. Air within the bladder's lumen. If this patient had contrast within the bowel and bladder on this scan, it would have the characteristic triad

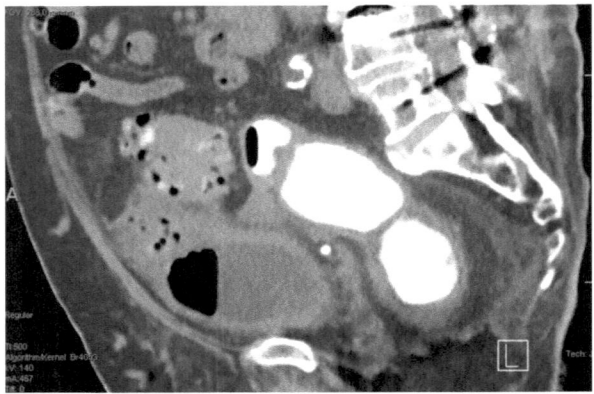

In the industrialized world, the leading cause of VV fistula formation is due to iatrogenic injury (75%). This is in contrast to a leading obstetric etiology in Africa, Asia, and South America. Risk factors for obstetric fistula formation during delivery include first marriage, socioeconomic status, short stature, and loss of follow-up with antenatal care. The exact worldwide prevalence of VV fistulas is unknown due to inadequate epidemiologic studies; however, it is thought to occur less than 1% following hysterectomy [20].

Vesicoenteric fistulas are characterized by the intestinal segment that is involved. They are either a colovesical fistula, rectovesical fistula, ileovesical fistula, and lastly appendico-vesical fistula. The most common vesicoenteric fistula is the colovesical fistula. [21]. This usually occurs at the bladder dome with connection to the sigmoid colon. The most common etiology of a colovesical fistula is diverticular disease (50–70%), reportedly occurring in 2% of all patients with diverticular disease. Colovesical fistula is three times more frequent in males than females [20].

5.8.2   Clinical Presentation

Iatrogenic fistulas tend to have a delayed presentation from the date of injury. Following surgery, only approx. 15% of patients will have symptoms within 1 month, while the majority will typically take months to develop. With radiation treatment, the disease process is even more delayed typically taking years until symptom onset [21] (see Fig. 5.22).

VV fistulas will result in urinary incontinence (see Fig. 5.23). This incontinence is typically continuous, as the tract is above the urethral outlet, but can become more pronounced following increases in abdominal pressure (ex: exercise). Patients who have had a gynecologic or intestinal surgery that had hematuria postoperatively should be assessed for possible urologic tract involvement/injury (see Fig. 5.24).

Initial symptomatology of vesicoenteric fistulas include lower urinary tract symptoms suggestive of infection (see Fig. 5.25). These include suprapubic pain,

Fig. 5.22 Cystoscopy, of the same patient in the above radiograph images, demonstrated a fistula os on the base/floor of the bladder. The os can be seen at 6 o'clock. (Vesicovaginal fistula)

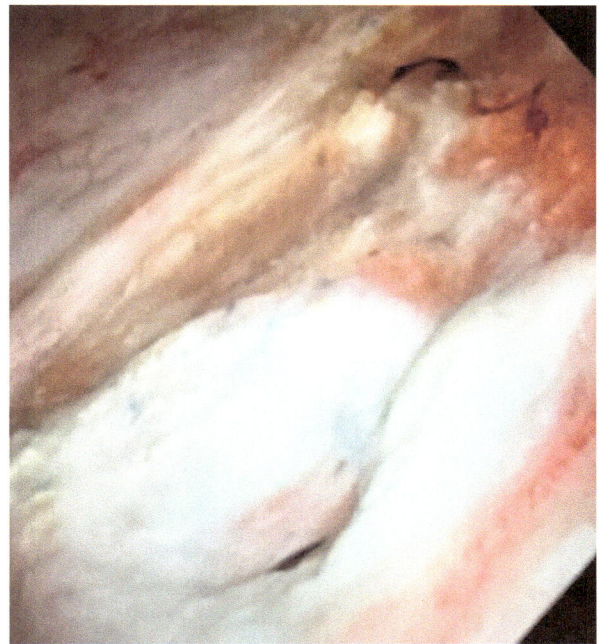

Fig. 5.23 The same os under closer cystoscopic inspection. The patient was noted to initially have a chief complaint of persistent urinary incontinence. The etiology of the fistula is presumed to be secondary to prior radiation therapy for cervical cancer. (Vesicovaginal fistula)

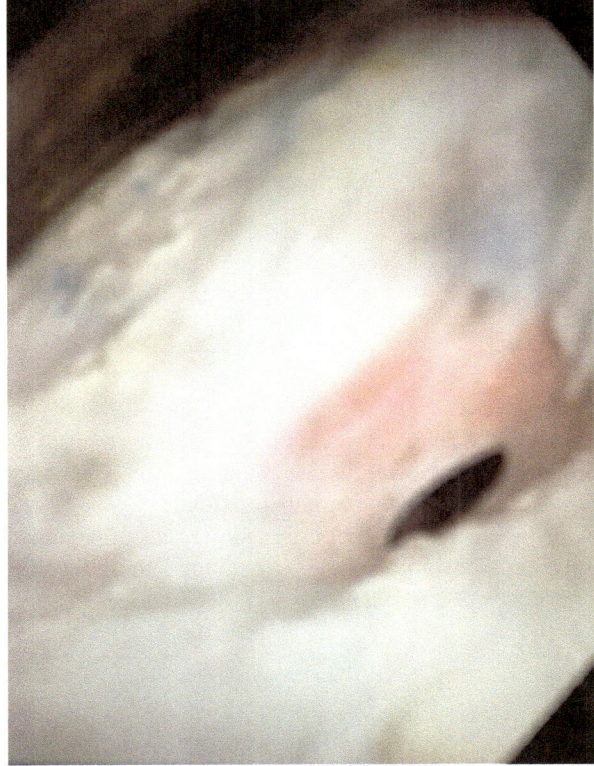

Fig. 5.24 Posterior right wall with evident large fistula os with protruding mucus. This vesico-cutaneous fistula resulted from a motor vehicle accident with an unidentified bladder injury months prior to presentation at our local hospital

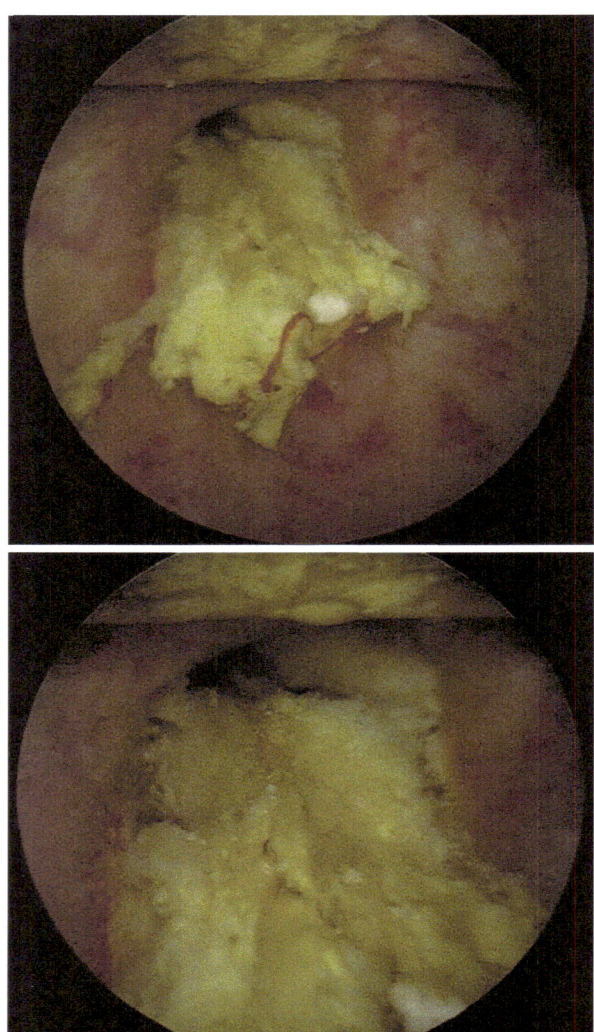

dysuria, frequency, and tenesmus (Gouverneur syndrome). Pneumaturia and fecaluria tend to be reported with larger fistulous tracts. Pneumaturia is more common in inflammatory bowel disease rather than malignancy. It is present 50 to 60% of the time and is not pathognomonic. This is explained to be caused by certain bacteria causing air with infection that may result in pneumaturia with no fistulous tract is present. Fecaluria however is pathognomonic for this condition and has a reported incidence of approximately 40% [21].

Fig. 5.25 Prominent area of erythema and bullous edema. This was found in a patient with feculent urine and suspected CV fistula. There was *no identified os with this fistula;* however, this was attributed to the markedly thickened and inflamed bladder wall. Contrasted imaging confirmed connection between the posterior wall of the bladder and sigmoid colon

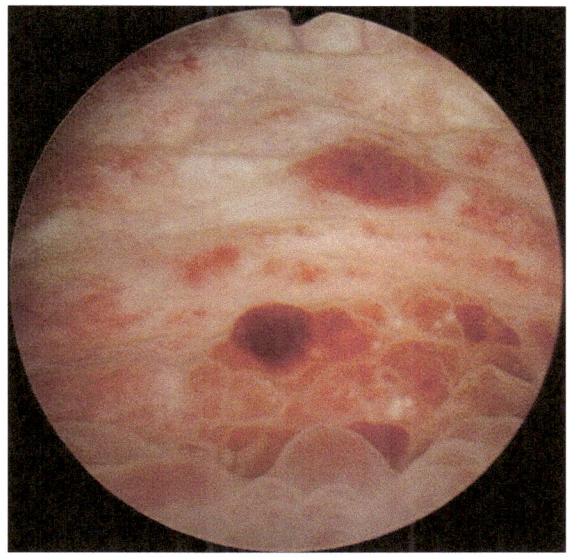

5.8.3 Cystoscopic Image(s)

5.8.4 Suggested Treatments

Cystoscopy of the bladder contributes to prevention, diagnosis, and treatment of the urogenital fistulous tract. When performing cystoscopy, the clinician should notate the size of the fistula os, the location of the os, and its relation to the vaginal stump, trigone, and ureteral orifices. The majority of post-hysterectomy fistulous tracts occur posterior to the inter-ureteral line and on the anterior vaginal wall. Pelvic examination with a speculum should always be performed in the evaluation of VVF. As with cystoscopy, the location, number, and size should be recorded precisely.

Cystoscopic findings for a vesicoenteric fistula will include identification of the os with associated localized bladder wall edema and congestion. There is bullous edema and perilesional mucosal hyperplasia and mature tracts. Suspicion should be high whenever feces or mucus is identified in the bladder as the os is not always readily identified. The lesions are frequently located at the level of the bladder dome. Role cystoscopy is additionally important because not only does it have a diagnosis but also allows for biopsy of the lesion.

Laboratory examination should include urinalysis and urine culture. Severe urinary tract infections should be treated; however, it should be reminded that with large enterovesical fistulas, sterilization of the urine is nearly impossible and sole conservative treatment may result in more virulent resistant pathogens.

Diagnostic radiographs are also very useful and may help to disclose a fistula tract that was missed upon cystoscopy. This is done by evident extravasation of contrast outside the bladder. Radiographs are also performed during cystoscopy with retrograde instillation of contrast to opacify the distal portions of the ureter. This is typically performed bilaterally, even if the os is lateralized, to rule out involvement of both ureters. Abdominal and pelvic CT is the most sensitive diagnostic method for colovesical fistulas. CT findings will demonstrate either intravesical air or extravasation of a contrast agent, thickened bladder wall possibly adjacent to loop of bowel, and presence of colonic diverticula.

The "double contrast" test is an old test used to differentiate between a vesicovaginal and a ureterovaginal fistula in the female patient. The test involves administering oral phenazopyridine and intravesical methylene blue while the patient has a tampon in her vagina. If the tampon turns orange a ureterovesical fistula is suspected. If the tampon turns blue, then a VV fistula is suspected. If the tampon has a mix of orange and blue, then suspicion for a complex fistula involving the ureters and bladder should be suspected [22].

The poppyseed test is an old but proven diagnostic test for enterovesical fistulas. Consisting of ingestion of a small quantity of poppy seeds, literature suggesting approx. 8 ounces, with a follow up analysis for the presence of poppy seeds in the urine in approximately 48 hours. Efficacy is reported to be comparable to CT scans (96% and 100% sensitivity and specificity respectively) [23].

Conservative management of urologic fistulas should only be performed for small tracts adequately characterized by cystoscopy or radiography. This will include urinary diversion/drainage via placement of a Foley catheter for 4–6 weeks, administration of antibiotics, and lastly measures directed at the involved non-urologic organs. Consideration for intravaginal conjugated estrogen to increase flexibility and rejuvenation of the vaginal wall for VV situlas or bowel rests with parental nutrition for vesicoenteric fistula.

Open surgery is the gold standard and most definitive intervention for patients with a urologic fistula. Surgically, most VV fistulas are repaired via a transvaginal approach. Surgery for a VV fustula can be instituted as early as 2–3 weeks after identification or after a waiting period of 2–3 months [21].

As with vesicovaginal fistulas the open surgical approach is the standard treatment with the most definitive outcomes for vesicoenteric fistulas. Surgery is either a one-stage or two-stage approach (colostomy with plans for reconstitution of bowel continuity once inflammation has decreased), which is primarily contingent on the severity of contamination of the bladder or pelvis.

Endoscopic treatment of fistulous tracts is limited. A small punctiform fistula os can undergo fulguration of the site with catheter drainage for 4–6 weeks. Radiographs or cystoscopy should be performed at the time of catheter removal to assess for adequate treatment.

Summary Key Points
- The most common site of urogenital fistula is between the bladder and the vagina, termed vesicovaginal fistulas (VV fistula). Other fistulas include vesicoenteric (intestinal tract) and less commonly vesicouterine (uterus).

  - In the North America and Europe, the leading cause of VV fistula is iatrogenic injury (approx. 75%). In Africa, Asia, and South America it is secondary to obstetrics.
  - Vesicoenteric fistulas are characterized by the intestinal segment that is involved: colovesical fistula (most common), rectovesical fistula, ileovesical fistula, and lastly appendico-vesical fistula.

- Symptomatology:

  - VV fistulas are likely to result in incontinence, this is guaranteed if the fistulous tract is superior to the sphincter. Incontinence can range from persistent to stress induced.
  - Vesicoenteric fistulas are associated with symptoms of urinary tract infection. Pneumaturia and fecaluria are likely to occur with large fistulous tracts. Fecaluria is pathognomonic.

    Gouverneur syndrome: suprapubic pain, dysuria, frequency, and tenesmus.

- Diagnostics:

  - Vesicovaginal fistula: Thorough physical exam including pelvic exam with speculum. The presence of a VVF can be confirmed by filling the bladder with dyed saline and observing for leakage. "Double contrast" test helps to differentiate between vesical versus ureteral involvement. VCUG is helpful but may fail to identify small fistulas. Cystoscopy is helpful to rule out an etiology of malignancy. It is important to document ostium/fistulous tract relation to ureters as this has surgical implications.
  - Vesicoenteric fistulas: CT of the abdomen and pelvis will demonstrate either intravesical air or extravasation of contrast agent, thickened bladder wall adjacent to a loop of bowel, and possibly the presence of colonic diverticula. Poppyseed test has a 96% sensitivity and 100% specificity. VCUG may be helpful. Colonoscopy/barium enema to exclude malignancy etiology.

- *Cystoscopic appearance:* Fistulas will have an ostium within the bladder. Sometimes the os is hidden behind extensive bullous mucosal edema. Fecaluria is pathognomonic. VVF tend to occur along the base of the bladder. Locations are the involved extra-genitourinary organs.
- Treatment: Endoscopic treatment limited. Punctiform os may be fulgurated with catheter placement to assist with healing. Otherwise, the majority require open surgery.

Additional References for Consideration
- Campbell-Walsh-Wein Urology by Alan W. Partin MD, PhD, Roger R. Dmochowski D, MMHC, FACS, Louis R. Kavoussi MD, MBA, and Craig A. Peters M
- Endoscopic Diagnosis and Treatment in Urinary Bladder Pathology by Petrisor A. Geavlete MD.

5.9   Bladder Lithiasis

5.9.1   Pathophysiology

Stone formation in the urologic tract occurs due to supersaturation/concentrated urine, with resultant crystal formation, and crystal aggregation (see Figs. 5.26, 5.27, and 5.28). This pathophysiologic process is assisted by a decrease in urinary stone

Fig. 5.26 Large bladder stone, measuring approximately 3.5 cm on radiographic imaging. Developed secondary to long-standing urinary retention from benign prostatic hyperplasia

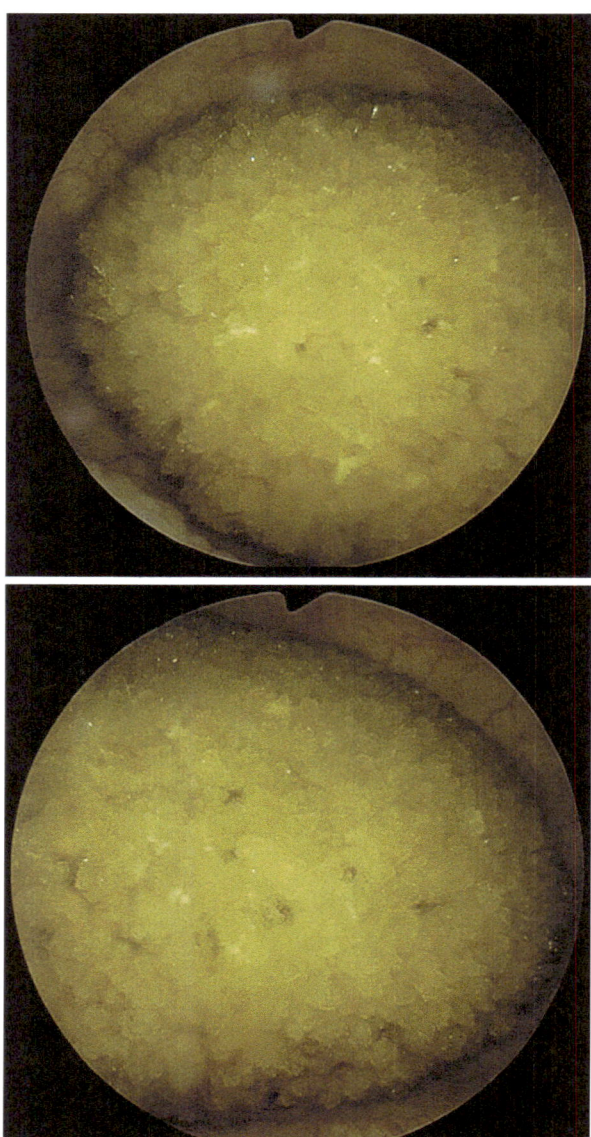

inhibitors (urinary citrate, urinary magnesium, Tamm-Horsfall proteins), and an increase in urinary stone promoters (high urine oxalate, low urine volume, cellular matrix, and epitaxy/cascade of crystal formation). Patient factors such as incomplete voiding, either secondary to an outlet obstruction or diminished contractility of the bladder, nearly always need to be present for stone formation to occur in the bladder.

Fig. 5.27 Large solitary bladder stone

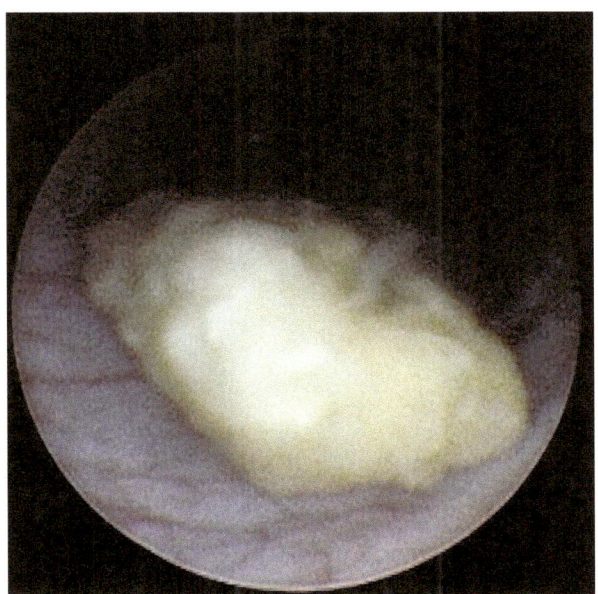

Fig. 5.28 Large solitary bladder stone with smooth surface

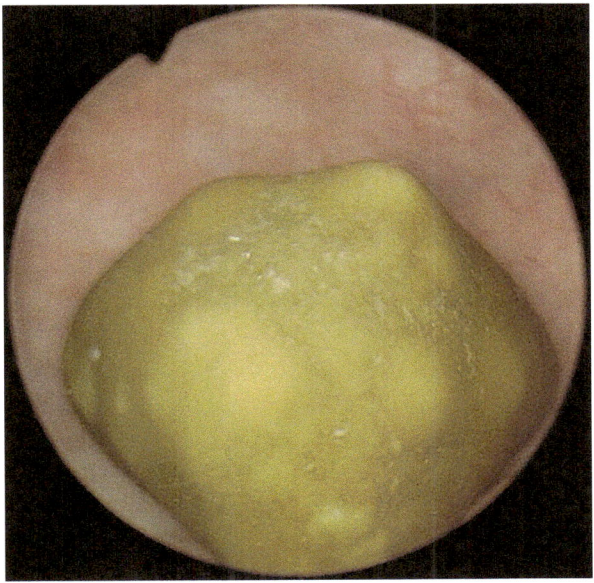

Studies have concluded that in approx. 80% of patients with bladder stones there is an associated outlet obstruction [24]. This is somewhat attributed to a higher prevalence of bladder stone formation in males than in females. In females, bladder stones typically occur due to urinary stasis from a cystocele or diverticulum rather than an outlet obstruction.

Impaired contractility resulting in urinary stasis is also known to result in stone formation. Patients who have had a spinal cord injury have a reported bladder stone incidence of approx. 15% [25]. Furthermore, the possible requirement for lifelong indwelling bladder drainage, with a catheter, contributes to this risk of bladder stone formation.

5.9.2   Clinical Presentation

Patients with bladder stones will present with symptoms of incomplete bladder emptying. In the sensate patient this will either be reported as increased frequency, inability to urinate or maintain stream, straining to urine, and dysuria. Patients with a spinal cord injury may not endorse lower urinary tract symptoms but may report issues with catheterization or malfunction of their indwelling Foley.

Laboratory workup should include a urinalysis and urine culture. The urinalysis will demonstrate significant hematuria, >5 RBCs, and may even be identified on gross examination. Terminal hematuria with a sudden cessation in voiding is the most common presentation for bladder calculi [26].

Diagnosis of a bladder stone is made by an abdominal pelvic radiograph. A standard "KUB" x-ray (kidney, ureter, and bladder film) should easily be able to identify a bladder stone. Patient body habitus, contractures, or musculoskeletal hardware may make for difficult interpretation of a KUB, and in this setting a low-dose non-contrasted CT scan is warranted. An ultrasound of the bladder is another alternative.

5.9.3   Cystoscopic Image(s)

5.9.4   Suggested Treatments

Endoscopic treatment is the first therapeutic option for bladder stones. This will consist of cystoscopic lithotripsy, termed cystolitholapaxy, utilizing either mechanical, ultrasound, or laser energy. Limitations to the endoscopic approach include very large and dense stones, numerous calculi, small caliber urethra, and a diminished bladder compliance for evacuation of the fragments.

Percutaneous surgery for large bladder stones is a second-line intervention for bladder stones, although extracorporeal shock wave lithotripsy has documented use as well. Indications for an open cystolithotomy include contraindications for transurethral or percutaneous approach such as small capacity bladders or severe urethral stricture disease [27].

Summary Key Points

- Stone formation occurs due to supersaturation/concentrated urine, with resultant crystal formation, and crystal aggregation. This is facilitated by decrease in urinary stone inhibitors and an increase in promoters.

  – Nearly all patients with bladder stone formation have associated outlet obstruction.

- Patients will present with obstructive urologic symptoms or have impaired bladder contractility leading to urinary retention.

  – Terminal hematuria with a sudden stop in voiding is a very common complaint.

- Diagnostics: UA will likely have significant microscopic hematuria. There will be crystals on analysis. KUB x-ray will readily identify the intravesical stone. Low dose noncontrast CT scan is an alternative to KUB.
- *Cystoscopic appearance*: Bladder stones vary in appearance: with differing color and size. They can range from yellow, to orange, to brown, and can be smooth or spiculated.
- Treatment: Endoscopic treatment is the first therapeutic option for bladder stones. Limitations include very large and dense stones, numerous calculi, small caliber urethra, and a diminished bladder compliance for evacuation of the fragments. Second-line interventions include percutaneous procedures or possibly open cystolithotomy.

Additional References for Consideration

- Penn Clinical Manual of Urology by Philip M. Hanno MD, MPH, Thomas J. Guzzo MD, MPH, S. Bruce Malkowicz MD and Alan J. Wein MD, FACS, PhD

5.10 Retained Foreign Bodies

5.10.1 *Pathophysiology*

A retained foreign body is any object that is left inside the patient by error, such as following a procedure or operation, and typically requires a subsequent procedure for removal [28]. Retained foreign bodies can also occur due to self-insertion for autoerotic purposes, result of penetrating wounds, and migration from other organs [29].

Retention of a device within the bladder or urethra predispose the patient to infection and urinary obstruction. Objects left within the urinary bladder can result in encrustation/stone formation.

5.10.2 Clinical Presentation

Patients who incidentally lose a self-inserted object within themselves should be able to present to the emergency department with a complaint of a retained foreign object. Patients who have undergone an anesthetized procedure with a medical device left in them may not be aware that a retained foreign body is present, unfortunately common with ureteral stents, although additionally due to loss of follow-up (see Figs. 5.29, 5.30, and 5.31). These patients will likely have a symptomatology of obstruction and urinary tract infection: dysuria, fevers/chills, flank pain, suprapubic pain, urinary frequency, and bladder spasms.

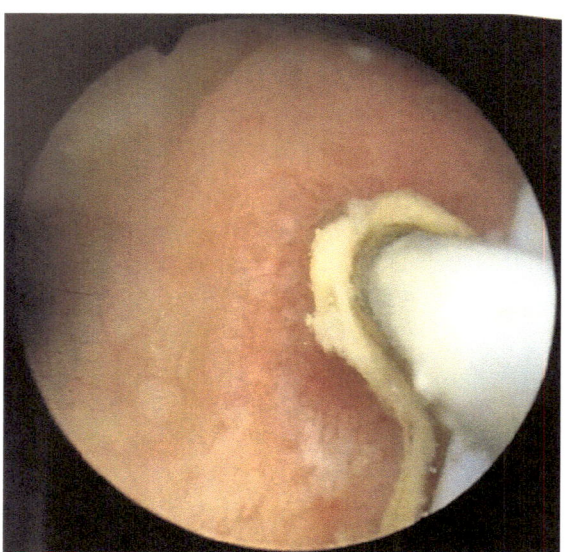

Fig. 5.29 Seen here is a retained right sided ureteral stent with significant encrustation in the bladder. The patient required laser lithotripsy of the encrusted stent and had a successful stent removal

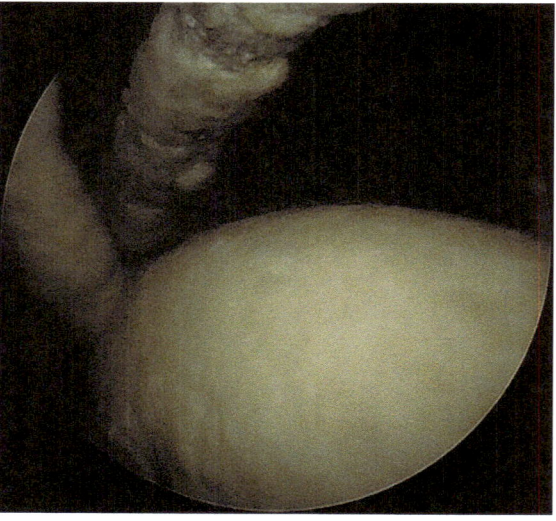

Fig. 5.30 Severely encrusted, 9-month-old, retained ureteral stent in pregnant patient. Stent was noted to have a dense 3 cm bladder stone attached to the distal curl

Fig. 5.31 Lateral wall of
the bladder with evident
Urolift metallic clip. The
therapeutic location of the
clip should be within the
prostatic urethra; clip
removed with resection
loop. Unknown on
migratory patterns of the
clip as the procedure was
performed by an outside
urologist

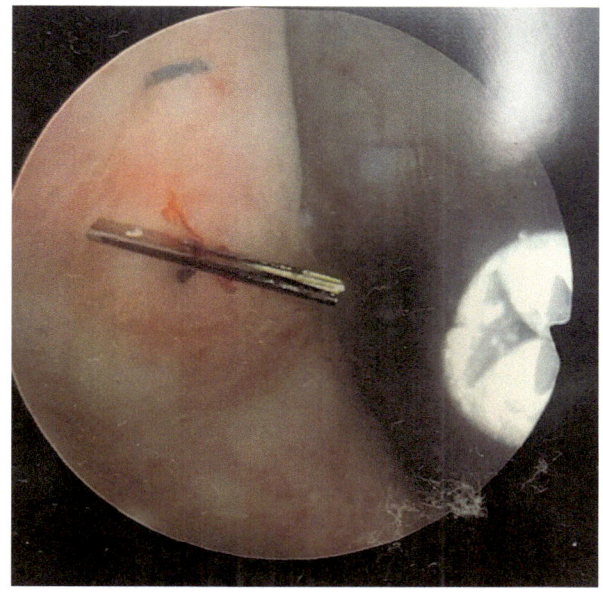

5.10.3   Cystoscopic Image(s)

5.10.4   Suggested Treatments

Treatment for retained foreign bodies involve removal of the offending object. This
will likely involve additional antibiotic administration prior and post procedure. If
device is significantly encrusted, this may require lithotripsy, as seen when performing a cystolitholapaxy.

Summary Key Points:
- A retained foreign body is any object that is accidentally left inside the patient,
  and typically requires a subsequent procedure for removal.
- Patients who incidentally lose a self-inserted object within themselves should be
  able to present to the emergency department with a complaint of a retained foreign object.

  – Alternatively, those unaware possibly 2/2 to surgical foreign body may pres-
    ent with UTI symptoms. Hopefully radiopaque and easily identifiable on x-ray.

- *Cystoscopic appearance:* Dependent upon the duration of the foreign body resid-
  ing in the bladder, there can be turbidity of urine and encrustation of the object.
- Treatment: Removal of the offending object with perioperative antibiotics.
  Encrusted objects will require cystolitholapaxy.

Additional References for Consideration
- Endoscopic Diagnosis and Treatment in Urinary Urethral Pathology by Petrisor
  A. Geavlete MD.
- Complications of Urologic Surgery by Samir S. Taneja MD, Ojas Shah MD

References

1. Hanno P. Lower urinary tract infections in women and pyelonephritis. In: Hanno P, Guzzo T, Malkowicz B, Wein A, editors. Penn clinical manual of urology. Philadelphia: Elsevier; 2021. p. 110–32.
2. Sabih A, Leslie S. Complicated urinary tract infections. In: Stat pearls. Treasure Island. Florida: StatPearls Publishing; 2021. Retrieved from https://pubmed.ncbi.nlm.nih.gov/28613784/.
3. Hanno P. Lower urinary tract infections in women and pyelonephritis. In: Hanno IP, editor. Penn clinical manual of urology. Saunders; 2014a. p. 110–32.
4. American Urological Association. (2021a). Nephrogenic Adenoma. Retrieved from AUA net: https://www.auanet.org/education/auauniversity/education-products-and-resources/pathology-for-urologists/urinary-bladder/non-neoplastic-lesions/nephrogenic-adenoma
5. American Urological Association. (2021b). Cystitis Glandularis. Retrieved from AUA net: https://www.auanet.org/education/auauniversity/education-products-and-resources/pathology-for-urologists/urinary-bladder/non-neoplastic-lesions/cystitis-glandularis
6. American Urological Association. (2021c). Inverted Papilloma. Retrieved from AUA net: https://www.auanet.org/education/auauniversity/education-products-and-resources/pathology-for-urologists/urinary-bladder/non-invasive-urothelial
7. Khater N. Bladder leiomyoma: presentation, evaluation, and treatment. Arab J Urol. 2013;11(1):54–61.
8. Cheng L, Nascimento A, Neumann R, Nehra A, Cheville C, Ramnani D, et al. Hemangioma of the urinary bladder. Am Cancer Soc J. 2000;86(3):498–504.
9. Castilo P, Gregorio S, Alcaide J, Basan A, Barthel J. Bladder Neurofibroma: case report and bibliographic review. Archivos Espanoles de Urologia. 2006;59(9):899–901.
10. Arnold H, Bourseaux F, Brock N. Neuartige Krebs-Chemotherapeutika aus der Gruppe der zyklischen N-Lost-Phosphamidester. Naturwissenschaften. 1958;45(3):64–6.
11. Sheperd J, Pringle L, Barnett M, et al. Mesna versus hyperhydration for prevention of cyclophosphamide-induced hemorrhagic cystitis in bone marrow transplantation. J Clin Oncol. 1991;9(11):2016–9.
12. Corman J, McClure D, Pritchett R, et al. Treatment of radiation induced hemorrhagic cystitis with hyperbaric oxygen. J Urol. 2003;169(6):2200–2.
13. Bernhoff E, Tylden G, Kjerpeseth L, Gutteberg T, Hirsch H, Rinaldo C. Leflunomide inhibition of BK virus replication in renal tubular epithelial cells. J Virol. 2010;84(4):2150–6.
14. American Urological Association. (2021d). Squamous Metaplasia. Retrieved from AUA net: https://www.auanet.org/education/auauniversity/education-products-and-resources/pathology-for-urologists/urinary-bladder/non-neoplastic-lesions/squamous-metaplasia
15. Moldwin R, Hanno P. Interstitial cystitis/bladder pain syndrome and related disorders. In: Partin A, Dmochowski R, Kavoussi L, Peters C, editors. Campbell-Walsh-Wein urology. Philadelphia: Elsevier; 2021. p. 1224–50.
16. Hanno P. Interstitial cystitis/bladder pain syndrome. In: Hanno P, Guzzo T, Malkowicz B, editors. Penn clinical manual of urology. Philadelphia: Saunders; 2014b. p. 195–200.
17. Whitmore K, Fall M, Sengiku A, Tomoe H, Logadottir Y, Ho Kim Y. Hunner lesion versus non-Hunner lesion interstitial cystitis/bladder pain syndrome. Int J Urol. 2019;26(1):26–34.
18. Oyama I, Rejba A, Lukban J, al, e. Thiele massage as therapeutic intervention for femal patients with interstitial cystitis and high tone pelvic floor dysfunction. Urology. 2004;64(5):862–5.
19. Gosling JA, Dixon J. Structure of trabeculated detrusor smooth muscle in cases of prostatic hypertrophy. Urol Int. 1980;35(5):351–5.
20. Smith A, Rovner E. Urinary fistula. In: Hanno P, Guzzo T, Malkowics B, Wein A, editors. Penn clinical manual of urology. Philadelphia: Saunders; 2014. p. 301–3018.
21. Geavlete P, Nita G, Dragutescu M, Mirciulescu V, Geavlete B. Endoscopic management of vescial fistulas. In: Geavlete P, editor. Endoscopic diagnosis and treatment in urinary bladder pathology. London: Elsevier; 2016. p. 277–91.

22. O'Brien W, Lynch J. Simplification of double-dye test to diagnose various types of vaginal fistulas. Urology. 1990;36(5):456.
23. Melchior S, Cudovic D, Jones J, Thomas C, Gillitzer R, Thuroff J. Diagnosis and surgical management of colovesical fistulas due to sigmoid diverticulitis. J Urol. 2009;182:978–82.
24. Douenias E, Rich M, Badlani G, et al. Predisposing factors in bladder calculi: review of 100 cases. Urology. 1991;37:240–3.
25. Lightner D. Contemporary urologic Management of Patients with Spincal cord injury. Mayo Clin Proc. 1998;73(5):434–8.
26. Leslie SW, Sajjad, H (2021, Sept 17). Bladder stones. Retrieved from In: StatPearls: https://www.ncbi.nlm.nih.gov/books/NBK441944/
27. Miller D. Percutaneous Nephrolithotomy using the laparoscopic entrapment sac. Urology. 2003;62:333–6.
28. Zejnullahu V, Bicaj B, Zejnullahu V, Hamza A. Retained surgical foreign bodies after surgery. Open Acc Macedonian J Med Sci. 2017;5(1):97–100.
29. Eckford S, Persad R, Brewster S, Gingell J. Intravesical foreign bodies: five-year review. Br J Urol. 1992;69(1):41–5.

Chapter 6
Malignant Bladder Pathology

6.1 Carcinoma In Situ

6.1.1 Pathophysiology

Carcinoma in situ, referred to as "CIS," of the bladder is a type of nonmuscle-invasive bladder cancer, accounting for roughly 10% of all non-detrusor muscle-involved tumors [1] (see Figs. 6.1, 6.2, 6.3, 6.4, and 6.5). CIS is a dysplastic process of the urothelium/mucosa/the most superficial layer of the bladder. Histologic examination will demonstrate severe irregular cellular structure and nuclear pleomorphism, but there is no invasion into the lamina propria (photo for histology). Nuclear pleomorphism is any marked variation in size, shape, and staining of the cell's nucleus.

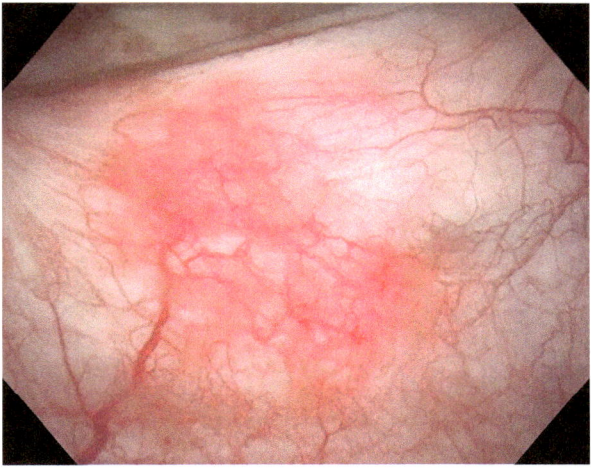

Fig. 6.1 Pictured above is an image of carcinoma in situ along the bladder base/trigone

B. C. Tenny, M. O'Neill, *Diagnostic Cystoscopy*,
https://doi.org/10.1007/978-3-031-10668-2_6

Fig. 6.2 An additional image of the same patient with carcinoma in situ along the bladder base/ trigone

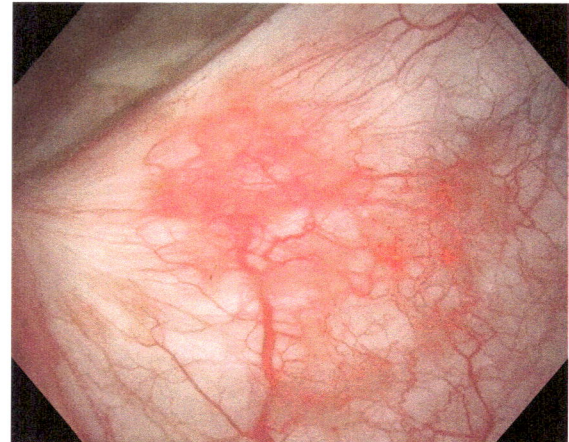

Fig. 6.3 Pictured is a solitary carcinoma in situ lesion along the posterior bladder wall seen under narrow band imaging. Pathology on TURBT demonstrated: Urothelial carcinoma in situ, negative for lamina propria invasion, muscularis propria is representative and negative for carcinoma. Lymph-vascular invasion is also not identified

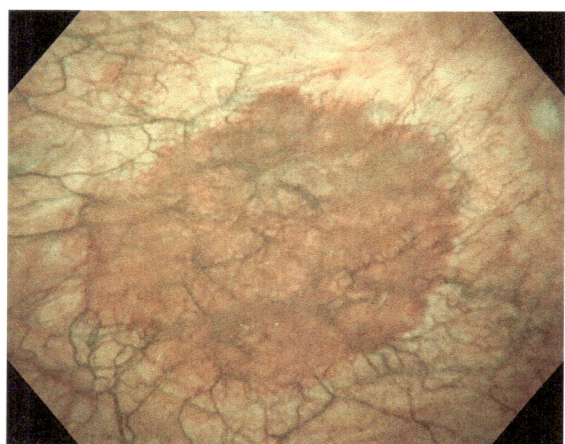

Fig. 6.4 Carcinoma in situ seen again, zoomed in, characterized by an erythematous well circumscribed lesion of the bladder

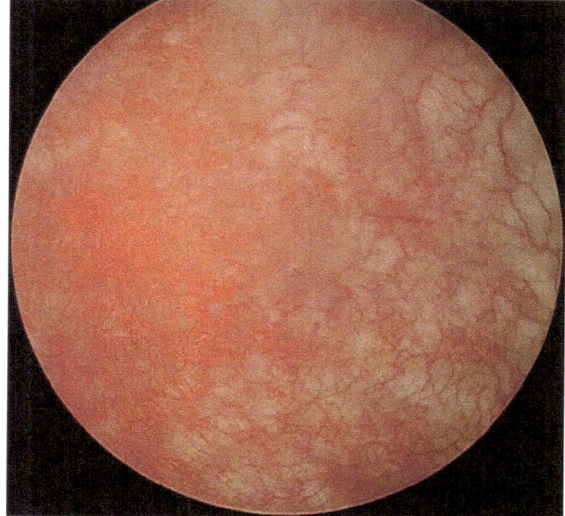

Fig. 6.5 Retroflexion assessment of the bladder neck with evident carcinoma in situ

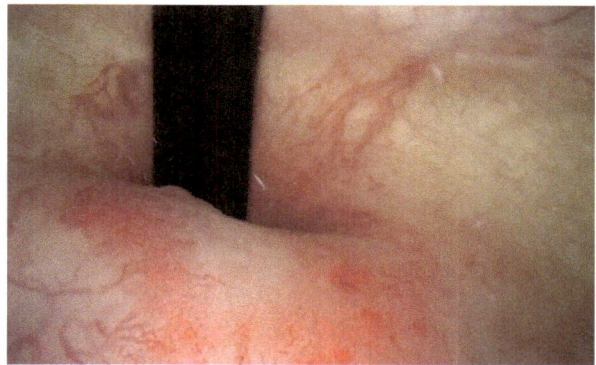

CIS, as it pertains to the bladder, is a high grade pathology with common reoccurrence in patients post endoscopic treatment, and a documented risk of progression to muscle invasion in >50% of cases [2]. Patients may have multiple lesions of low grade bladder cancer along with CIS, but the mere presence of CIS warrants a high-risk stratification. Treatment for bladder tumors is based upon the stratified risk of the tumor to progress to muscle invasion.

6.1.2   Clinical Presentation

Painless hematuria is the most common reported symptom of noninvasive bladder tumors. CIS differs in that there can also be reports of irritative voiding symptoms. In fact, certain studies report up to approx. 80% of CIS cases endorsing some irritative lower urinary tract symptoms [3]. Diagnosis is thus imperative because of the nonspecific symptomatology. Hematuria is a red flag for bladder cancer and warrants diagnostic cystoscopy.

Furthermore, patients who present with hematuria should additionally have a urine cytology and CT "Urogram" performed per hematuria AUA guidelines. Urine cytology is highly specific for high grade bladder cancer; in fact, studies have shown that a persistently positive urine cytology predicts the occurrence of high grade urinary tract cancer within 24 months, while radiography and cystoscopy may be negative [4]. Meaning, if the urine cytology for a patient is positive, there exists a high likelihood that they have cancer. The sensitivity of the test is "poor," as the test may miss low grade disease. Meaning, if the urine cytology is negative there may remain a tumor within the patient.

6.1.3 Cystoscopic Image(s)

6.1.4 Suggested Treatments

Surgical treatment of CIS is imperative. A transurethral resection of the bladder tumor under anesthesia is the initial treatment for any visible tumor and helps to identify the culprit lesion once the pathology has returned. A repeat resection is typically performed at 6 weeks, per AUA guidelines, to ensure no progression of tumor or that an incomplete resection was performed. To illustrate the importance, studies have shown upstaging on pathology in approx. 30% of repeat resections [5].

Post-resection intravesical therapy involves the administration of chemotherapy to annihilate freely floating tumor cells, preventing implantation along new walls/areas of the bladder. This therapy has greater efficacy low grade disease. CIS is a high grade pathology. BCG is never used post TUR due to the risk of systemic absorption, and all chemotherapy is contraindicated in cases with concern for perforation.

BCG, Bacille Calmette-Guerin, is an attenuated mycobacterium vaccine. It is reconstituted with sterile saline and administered into the bladder for intravesical immunotherapy. Therapy is initiated approx. 1 month post tumor resection, allowing for healing of the resection bed, and a urinalysis should be performed earlier to ensure no significant bleeding nor infection is occurring. Instillation dwell intervals last from 1–2 h.

BCG has a robust tumor-free response rate for CIS; initial responses are around 80% [6]. And 50% of those responses will continue to have a durable tumor-free rate for 4 years. This tumor-free rate continues to decline to approx. 30% at 10 years post treatment. Of the 70% that do reoccur following BCG, the majority relapse within the first 5 years. Currently the AUA recommends BCG as the preferred first line treatment option for high-risk bladder tumors, which includes CIS [7].

Intravesical chemotherapy is an alternative to BCG treatment; however, the rates of progression and reoccurrence are not as robust as immunotherapy. Intravesical chemotherapy may be preferred over immunotherapy if there are contraindications to BCG: immunocompromised, hx of BCG sepsis, gross hematuria due to extravasation risk, urinary tract infection (relative contraindication), and post TURBT [7].

Cystectomy, photodynamic therapy, radiation therapy, or systemic therapy is indicated in CIS cases for patients who fail BCG therapy. Failure is defined as either recurrent or persistent disease following a 6-week course of immunotherapy. Of those with a reoccurrence following the first treatment, a second course results in a 30–50% response rate [8]. Declaring failure should be a slow process up to 6 months post treatment, as studies have deemed a rising tumor-free response rate from approx. 50% to 80% 3–6 months after therapy [9].

In patients who have sole CIS, without any other tumors present, and have undergone cystectomy, up to 20% are found to have muscle invasion, upstaging, on final pathology of the bladder [10].

CIS is a high grade nonmuscle-invasive type of urothelial bladder cancer.

Summary Key Points

- CIS is a high grade nonmuscle-invasive type of urothelial bladder cancer. Risk of reoccurrence with endoscopic procedures alone is common, and there is documented risk of progression in at least 50% of cases.
- Patients may present with a gross or microscopic hematuria. CIS can cause irritative voiding symptoms (80% prevalence).
- Diagnosis of CIS is facilitated by cystoscopy and urine cytology. Urine cytology is highly specific for high grade bladder cancer, including CIS.
- *Cystoscopic appearance:* CIS will have a flat erythematous appearance, typically with easily demarcated borders.
- Treatment: Treatment for CIS first includes TURBT with repeat resection in 6 weeks. This ensures no progression of tumor (approx. 30%) or that incomplete resection occurred.

  - Post TURBT, CIS is responsive to BCG therapy (80% initial response with 50% of those patients lasting for 4 years, and 30% at 10 years). Most reoccurrence happens with 5 years post therapy.
  - BCG should be tried twice, as the second course has a tumor-free response rate of 30–50%. Declaring failure should be delayed until 6 months post treatment.
  - Intravesical chemo is an appropriate alternative to BCG therapy. BCG contraindications include immunocompromised, hx of BCG sepsis, gross hematuria, UTI, and post TURBT.
  - BCG failure, and/or upstaging/progression on re-resection, may be best treated with cystectomy, photodynamic therapy, radiation therapy, or systemic therapy.

Additional References for Consideration

- Campbell-Walsh-Wein Urology by Alan W. Partin MD, PhD, Roger R. Dmochowski D, MMHC, FACS, Louis R. Kavoussi MD, MBA, and Craig A. Peters M
- Penn Clinical Manual of Urology by Philip M. Hanno MD, MPH, Thomas J. Guzzo MD, MPH, S. Bruce Malkowicz MD and Alan J. Wein MD, FACS, PhD
- Endoscopic Diagnosis and Treatment in Urinary Bladder Pathology by Petrisor A. Geavlete MD.

6.2 Bladder Cancer (Papillary and Sessile Lesions)

6.2.1 Pathophysiology

Bladder cancer is the fourth most common cancer in men; it is notably less common (not even the top ten) in women, but some studies have demonstrated a graver prognosis when diagnosed in females [11].

Urothelial bladder cancer can be divided by the pathologic grade into the following groups: CIS (previously discussed), papillary urothelial neoplasm of low malignant potential, low grade urothelial carcinoma, and lastly high grade urothelial cancer.

Papillary urothelial neoplasm of low malignant potential or PUNLMP is papillary growth with minimal cytologic atypia. Progression rates to high grade disease/muscle-invasive bladder cancer is reassuringly less than 1% [12]. Low grade urothelial carcinoma is characterized by some nuclear atypia and increased cellular size on histologic examination, and typically pedunculated formation on cystoscopic assessment (see Fig. 6.6). Low grade tumors frequently reoccur but reassuringly have a low progression to more advanced/high grade cancers after 5 years (48–71% reoccurrence and 2–12% progression rate) [13]. Low grade urothelial tumors are the most commonly encountered malignant bladder tumors approximating 50% [14].

High grade urothelial cancer has significant dysplastic features on histologic examination: disordered growth, significant nuclear atypia/numerous mitotic features present, and pleomorphic cells with exaggerated nuclei. These lesions are invasive/high risk for disease progression (25% risk of tumor stage progression). High grade urothelial cancer can be further stratified, for prognostic significance, by histology if there is a variant found. Common variants to high urothelial cancer are the following: micropapillary, sarcomatoid variant, plasmacytoid variant, nested variant, and divergent differentiation such as squamous or glandular differentiation (see Figs. 6.7 and 6.8).

Micropapillary, known since 1994, occurs approximately 0.7–2.2% in all UCC tumors [15], and is associated with a more progressive disease course. A study by Kamat et al. in [16] demonstrated that approximately 50% of cases are diagnosed

Fig. 6.6 Fulguration of a low grade TA tumor. Patient had known TA disease and underwent repeat cystoscopy in 3 months that confirmed reoccurrence. Tissue was sent for pathology that confirmed mucosal invasion

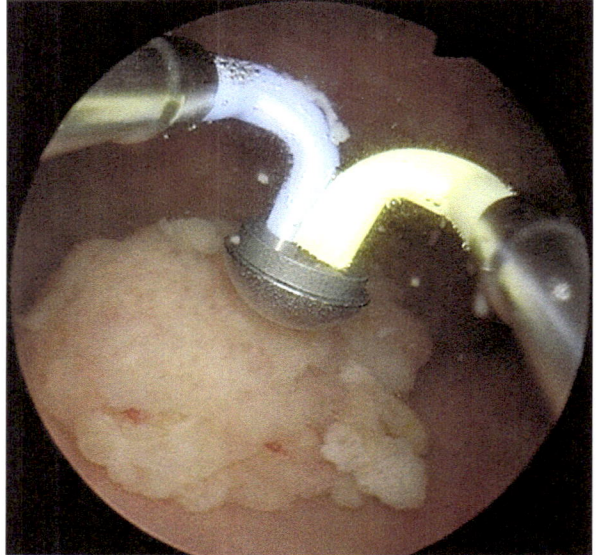

Fig. 6.7 Large pedunculated papillary tumor arising from the left lateral wall. Resection revealed high grade papillary urothelial carcinoma with a micropapillary variant. Tumor was noted to be invading into the muscularis propria; the patient was inevitably set up for a cystectomy

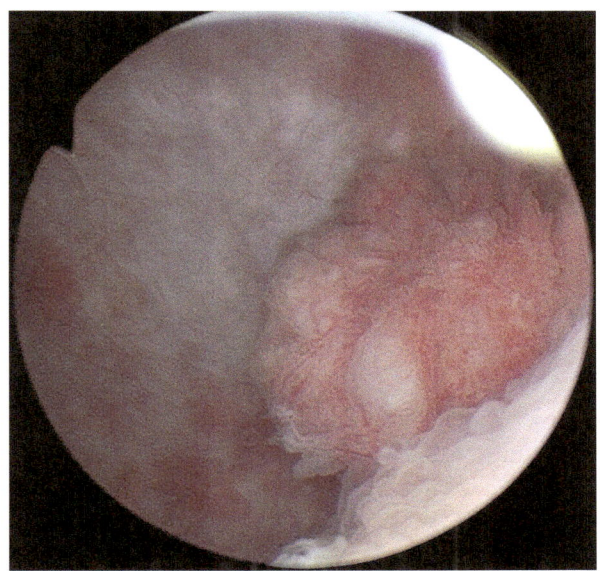

late in their clinical course, once T3 or T4 [16]. Sarcomatoid variant also have a low prevalence; nearly all variants do. The sarcomatoid variant tumors tend to be large infiltrative masses on diagnosis, and poorly respond to systemic chemotherapy. Plasmacytoid and nested variants are both rare, and like the other variants carry a grim prognosis.

Divergent differentiation means the tumor exhibits more than one line of progenitor cells [17]. Squamous differentiation is found in resected tumors approx. 16–22% of the time; however, may have an incidence of up to 60% [18]. Glandular differentiation comprises small gland-like spaces in typical urothelial carcinoma cells. It is found approx. 10% of the time. Glandular differentiation may be locally advanced on initial diagnosis, but evidence has demonstrated a similar rate of survival and recurrence-free life post treatment when compared to typical UCC [19].

Nonurothelial/nontransitional cell cancers are less common types of bladder cancer, and include small cell carcinoma (rare), squamous cell cancer, and adenocarcinoma. Small cell carcinoma is a neuroendocrine neoplasm that arises from nerve cells/neuroendocrine cells. Small cell cancer is clinically aggressive but fortunately sensitive to chemotherapy. Squamous cell carcinoma accounts for up to 5% of all bladder cancers [20], and its formation is associated with chronic inflammation. Adenocarcinoma arises from epithelial dysplasia with a pure glandular phenotype. Interestingly, secondary bladder adenocarcinoma is more prevalent than primary bladder adenocarcinoma, and thus it is important to rule out cancers elsewhere. Adenocarcinoma is not chemosensitive and thus surgical resection tends to be the mainstay [13].

Fig. 6.8 Multiple high grade bladder tumors in the same patient; found along the left lateral (above) and anterior walls (below). Histological assessment confirmed high grade urothelial carcinoma without lamina propria nor muscularis invasion. Patient diagnosed with high grade TA disease

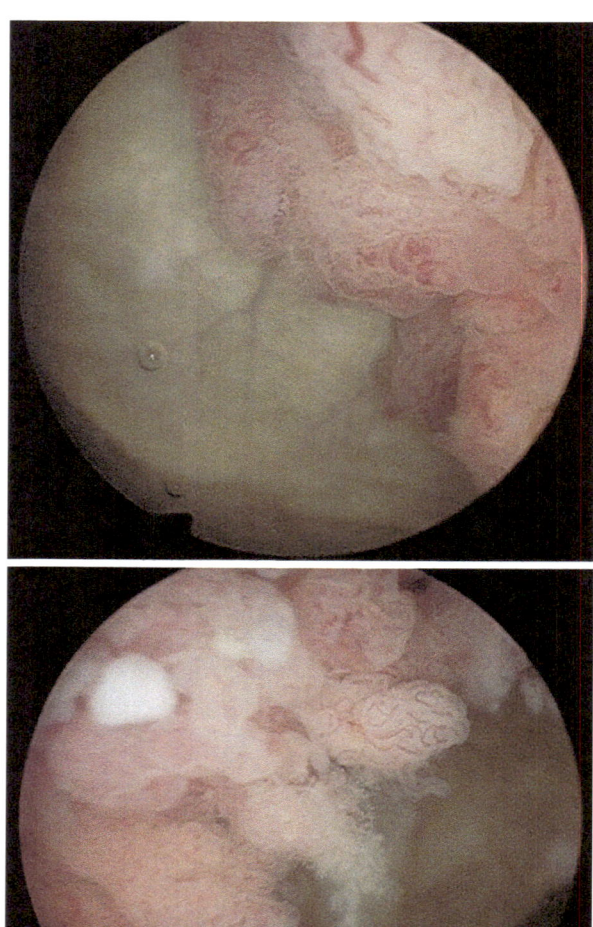

6.2.2   Clinical Presentation

The prototypical bladder cancer patient is a white male around the age of 70 (median age of diagnosis). Males have a reported 3-4x higher prevalence of bladder cancer than females, and the disease risk is twice as common in white males compared to their black counterparts.

Patients with bladder cancer may present with the following risk factors: a first degree relative for bladder cancer (yields a 2x increased risk for developing the disease), tobacco use (2-3x increased risk for bladder cancer), industrial exposure to aniline dyes or rubber manufacturing, infection of *Schistosoma haematobium* (common in parts of northern Africa), chronic irritation and inflammation, prior pelvic irradiation (associated with an approximate 10% increased risk of developing bladder cancer), and ingestion of the Chinese herb *Aristolochia fangchi*, phenacetin (antipyretic analgesic banned in the US around 1960), and lastly ochratoxin [14].

Chief signs and symptoms include hematuria, both microscopic and gross, dysuria, urinary frequency, sensation of incomplete emptying, and other irritative complaints. Hematuria is found in 85% of bladder cancer patients, and thus the presence of blood should warrant urologic evaluation. Bladder cancer is diagnosed by cystoscopy, urine cytology, and radiographic imaging (see Figs. 6.8, 6.9 and 6.10).

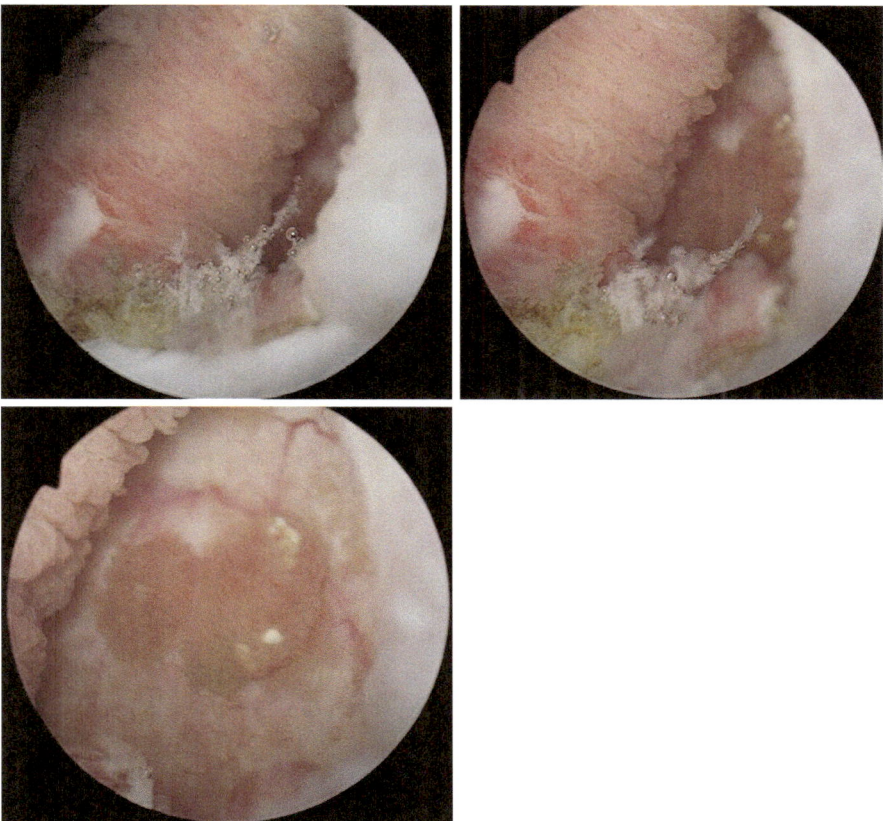

Fig. 6.9 Left lateral anterior wall with diverticula and evident small bladder tumors within. Histological review following resection demonstrated low grade urothelial carcinoma

Fig. 6.10 Large 2 cm
appearing right peri-
trigonal/ureteral orifice
bladder tumor. Tumors was
resected without
involvement of the
UO. Histologic
examination revealed low
grade papillary urothelial
carcinoma

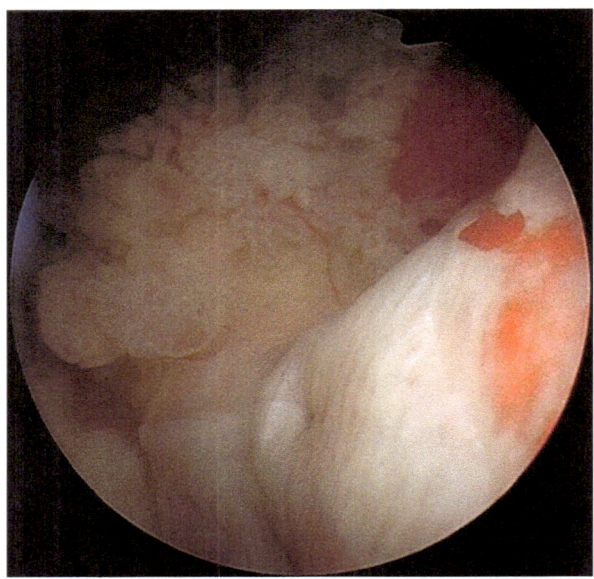

6.2.3 Cystoscopic Image(s)

6.2.4 Suggested Treatments

Treatment of bladder cancer is dependent upon the TNM stage and histologic type
found after transurethral resection (see Table 6.1). Post transurethral resection of a
known bladder cancer, the clinician can administer immediate intravesical chemotherapy to prevent reoccurrence. This therapy demonstrates a robust 39% reduction
in reoccurrence over the first following 2 years and works best with solitary Ta or
T1 tumors [14].

Low grade Ta disease can be treated by transurethral resection (TURBT) along
with perioperative intravesical instillation of chemotherapy. Cystoscopy is then performed routinely to assess for any recurrence (at out center we perform cystoscopy
every 3 months for the first 2 years, then every 6 months for the next 2 years, and
then 1 annual examination for 5 years post. A reoccurrence calls for a return to every
3-month cystoscopic assessment) (see Fig. 6.11). Small low grade reoccurrences
can be treated by office fulguration.

High grade Ta disease is also treated with TURBT and immediate intravesical
instillation. A second look cystoscopy TURBT is typically planned within approx.
6 weeks post to ensure that there was no missed T1 or higher disease. Upstaging
occurs on approx. 15% patients who initially had high grade Ta disease [22] If there
is no lamina propria or muscularis invasion on the second look cystoscopy, the typical treatment regimen consists of intravesical immunotherapy/BCG therapy. BCG is
started 2–4 weeks post tumor resection allowing for wound healing.

Table 6.1 The table incorporates data adapted from Steinberg [21]

Tumor		Lymph nodes		Metastasis	
TX	Primary tumor cannot be assessed	NX	Lymph nodes cannot be assessed		
T0	No evidence of primary tumor	N0	No lymph node metastasis	MO	No metastasis
Ta	Noninvasive papillary carcinoma. Limited to the mucosa.	N1	Single regional lymph node metastasis (in the true pelvis)	M1	Distant metastasis
Tis	Carcinoma in situ	N2	Multiple regional lymph node metastasis		
T1	Tumor invades lamina propria	N3	Lymph node metastasis to the common iliac lymph nodes		
T2	Tumor invades the muscularis propria				
T3	Tumor invades the perivesical tissue/fat (whole bladder involvement)				
T4	Tumor invades surrounding organs: prostate, seminal vesicles, uterus, vagina, pelvic wall, abdominal wall				

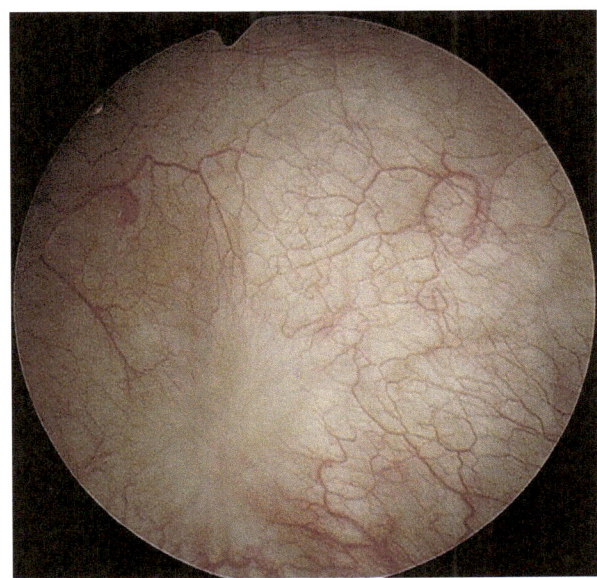

Fig. 6.11 No tumor present. Old resection scar seen at 7'o clock. Easily appreciated by the slight devascularization of the mucosa

T1 disease treated with initial TURBT should receive immediate intravesical chemotherapy. Studies have identified upstaging in 25% on the second look TURBT [23]. If there is no upstaging to muscle-invasive cancer, consideration should be given for BCG therapy versus "early" cystectomy (as in prior to disease progression). BCG efficacy in T1 bladder cancer can be assessed by the incidence of reoccurrence or progression of disease following therapy, 16–40% and 4.4–40% respectively [24]. Factors that decrease the efficacy of BCG therapy include multiple tumors, co-occurring CIS, individual tumors measuring larger than 3 cm [25]. Due to these clinical features demonstrating a divergence in patient outcomes/ natural history of the disease, patients with nonmuscle-invasive bladder cancer should undergo risk stratification for the determination of BCG therapy versus early cystectomy. Per the AUA guidelines, a patient with low grade T1 disease without variant histology and the aforementioned cystoscopic findings is intermediate risk. The clinician should consider a 6-week course of induction intravesical chemo or BCG. If said patient has a complete response to the induction therapy, he or she is to undergo maintenance therapy for 1 year (high risk disease requires maintenance therapy of 3 years following complete response). Partial responses to induction therapy warrant consideration for reattempt or proceeding with cystectomy. High risk patients who have a complete response to BCG should have maintenance therapy for 3 years [26].

T2 or greater bladder tumors will require surgical resection. Radical cystectomy is the standard of care for bladder cancer that invades into or through the bladder's muscle layer. Therefore, it is incredibly important to obtain the muscularis propria layer upon transurethral resection for adequate staging. With cystectomy, the patient will be given some form of urinary diversion. Urinary diversion ranges from ileal conduits, continent pouches, and orthotopic continent diversion. Lastly, any form of metastatic disease warrants systemic chemotherapy.

Summary Key Points
- Bladder cancer is most commonly a urothelial cell carcinoma. Within this type of cancer, there are both low malignant lesions and worrisome high grade tumors.

  - Low grade UCC tumors frequently reoccur (48–71%) and have a low rate of progression (approx. 2–10%). Low grade tumors make up 50% of all found bladder cancers.
  - High grade UCC tumors have a reported 25% risk of progression.
  - Variants and differentiation of UCC tumors may increase the likelihood of reoccurrence and progression.

- Chief signs and symptoms include hematuria, both microscopic and gross, dysuria, urinary frequency, sensation of incomplete emptying, and other irritative complaints. Hematuria is found in 85% of bladder cancer patients, and thus the presence of blood should warrant urologic evaluation.
- Diagnosis is facilitated by cystoscopy, urine cytology, and radiographic imaging (CT Urogram).
- *Cystoscopic appearance:* Tumor appearance can vary to a significant degree. Lesions can be pedunculated with a single stalk or be sessile as growing out from the mucosal floor. Sessile lesions tend be higher grade. Furthermore, the color and papillary appearance can suggest malignant potential.
- Preferred treatment is dictated by stage and grade of tumor:

  - Low grade Ta disease- > TURBT with periop intravesical chemo. Cystoscopy surveillance plan of q3–6 months for first 2 years, q6–9 months for the next 2

years, and then annually for the fifth year. Recurrence calls for starting the
cysto surveillance plan from the beginning.
- High grade Ta disease- > TURBT with periop intravesical chemo. Second
  look cysto in 6 weeks. If no progression, BCG therapy 2–4 weeks post TURBT.
- T1 disease- > TURBT with periop intravesical chemo. Second look cysto in
  6 weeks. If no progression, consider BCG versus early cystectomy. Can be
  further stratified into low grade and high grade groups. Tumor characteristics
  greatly affect outcome. Approx. 25% upstaging/progression rate.

  BCG therapy efficacy has a reported recurrence of 16–40% with similar
  progression rates.

- T2 disease- > Preferred treatment includes radical cystectomy with urinary
  diversion.

Additional References for Consideration
- Campbell-Walsh-Wein Urology by Alan W. Partin MD, PhD, Roger
  R. Dmochowski D, MMHC, FACS, Louis R. Kavoussi MD, MBA, and Craig
  A. Peters M
- Penn Clinical Manual of Urology by Philip M. Hanno MD, MPH, Thomas
  J. Guzzo MD, MPH, S. Bruce Malkowicz MD and Alan J. Wein MD, FACS, PhD
- Endoscopic Diagnosis and Treatment in Urinary Bladder Pathology by Petrisor
  A. Geavlete MD.

6.3 Extrinsic Malignant Invasion

6.3.1 Pathophysiology

Although uncommon and late into the disease course, cancer from surrounding
organs can invade into the bladder, staging the tumor as T4 (stage 4 cancer). The
most common implicated cancers are prostate cancer (addressed in the urethral
malignant section of this textbook), colorectal cancer, gynecologic cancers, and
sarcomas.

Colorectal cancer has a few histopathologic variants similar to other organs;
however, the vast majority (approx. 95%) are due to adenocarcinoma [27]. On
microscopic assessment, primary adenocarcinoma of the bladder may be indistin-
guishable from adenocarcinoma of the colorectum, thus requiring histology with an
immunopathological assay (see Fig. 6.12). It should be noted that invasion of
colorectal cancer into the bladder is more common than bladder cancer invading the
colon or rectum [28].

Gynecological cancer, either cervical cancer or uterine (typically endometrial
cancer) cancer, can invade into the bladder if the pathology is invasive and high
grade. Cervical cancer with bladder invasion accounts for only 1.7% of patients
with a cervical cancer diagnosis, and has demonstrated a 5-year survival of around

Fig. 6.12 Large invasive secondary bladder tumor found in a patient with known rectal cancer. CT scan was concerning invasion into the base of the bladder. Cystoscopy was performed as a part of hematuria (predominantly microscopic but intermittently gross) surveillance. Biopsy confirmed adenocarcinoma, gastrointestinal phenotype

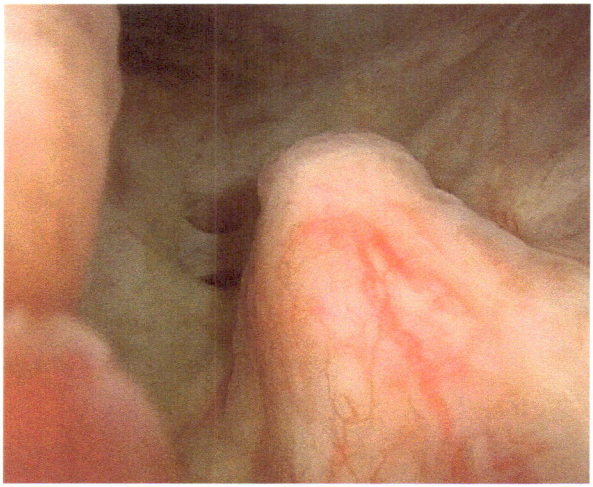

30% with irradiation and/or surgery [29]. Overall, endometrial carcinoma is typically believed to have a good prognosis, with approx. 80% not succumbing to the disease process. [30]. Those who have stage 4A disease, invading the bladder tends to have a five-year survival of around 17% [31].

Sarcoma, a tumor that arises from mesenchymal cells, is fortunately uncommon accounting for approximately 1% of all adult cancers [32]. Patients typically present late in the disease course due to relatively nonspecific symptoms until there is associated involvement of adjacent organs. Commonly, when the abdomen and pelvis are the sites for sarcoma growth, the gastrointestinal and urinary tract are displaced causing symptoms, and rarely this can result in local invasion. Early in their tumor growth cycle, the tumors are noted to be well encapsulated; however, after prolonged pressure and compression of adjacent organs, they tend to result in invasion [33].

6.3.2   Clinical Presentation

Nongenitourinary tumors that invade the bladder should be managed by a multidisciplinary team. Typically, the service that is associated with the primary cancer leads overall treatment planning with urologic consultation assisting. Patients may receive neoadjuvant or adjuvant therapies depending on the origin of the tumor. Overall survival is surprisingly moderate with a 3-year rate of about 40% [33].

Patients who have locally advanced tumors invading the bladder tend to have irritative lower urinary tract symptoms. This is secondary to the compression and direct infiltration of the bladder (see Fig. 6.13). Gross incontinence may demonstrate a fistulous tract that has formed due to the local invasion. Patient may also have hematuria, flank pain from obstruction of the upper urinary tract, and recurrent urinary tract infections.

Fig. 6.13 Pictured is the mass effect on the right posterior lateral wall of the bladder secondary to ovarian cancer. Large cystic dilation of the ovary causing distortion of the normal bladder contour. Fortunately, the was no invasion into the bladder as noted on MRI

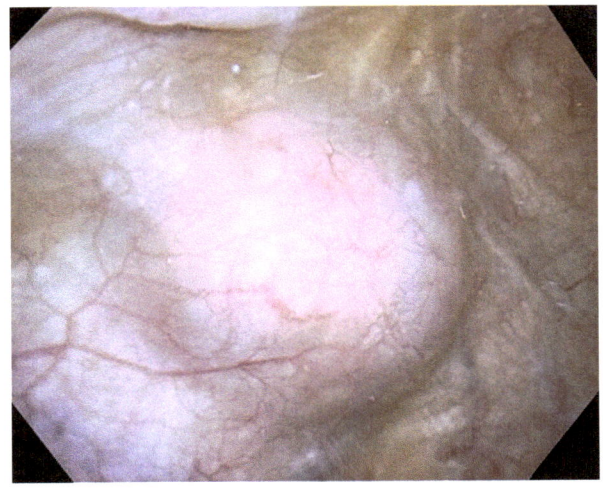

Diagnosis of either colorectal or gynecologic cancer invading the bladder is typically made by using radiographic imaging, cystoscopic assessment, and lastly either colonoscopy or gynecologic examination. In short, cystoscopy should always be performed for the evaluation of a lower urinary tract tumor.

MRI has been shown to exclude bladder or rectal involvement of cervical cancer with a specificity in the range of 88–91%; notably the MRI has a high negative predictive value but a lower positive predictive value [34]. This is due to its superior soft tissue contrast resolution.

6.3.3   Cystoscopic Image(s)

6.3.4   Suggested Treatments

Extirpative procedures for colorectal cancer invading the bladder can include partial and total bladder resections. Surgical outcomes for such resections are also not entirely poor if there is no other metastatic disease and surgical margins are negative. The decision for partial resection/bladder sparing procedure versus extreme total pelvic exenteration is dependent upon features of the primary tumor and patient. One study demonstrated a mean survival of 44 months following either partial or complete cystectomy for invasive colorectal cancer [35]. Furthermore, the consideration for neoadjuvant chemotherapy may assist in downsizing of the tumor and improve negative margins at the time of surgery.

Cervical cancer patients with bladder invasion will likely have irradiation as part of their treatment course along with chemotherapy; while exenteration is left for persistent disease post radiation treatment or recurrent central disease [29].

Furthermore, radiation in conjunction with chemotherapy has been reported to cure 40–50% of patients with recurrent disease following radical surgery [33].

For sarcomas, complete surgical resection is the only potentially curative treatment option, as local recurrence is responsible for approximately 75% of all sarcoma-related deaths [36]. Thus, frozen section should be performed to ensure complete resection at the time of surgery. Lastly, neoadjuvant chemotherapy and or radiation therapy may also be helpful in reducing local recurrence.

Summary Key Points
- Most common cancers with malignant invasion into the bladder are prostate cancer, colorectal cancer, gynecologic cancers (primarily cervical), and sarcomas.

  – Vast majority of colorectal cancers are primary adenocarcinoma.

- Presenting signs and symptoms will depend on the primary tumor. Expect bleeding from the primary organ system as well as a host of other constitutional symptoms: weight loss, fatigue, and abdominal or pelvic pain.
- Diagnosis is facilitated by workup of the primary tumor. MRI has shown superior imaging results in assessing for proximal soft tissue invasion. Cystoscopy should be performed for the evaluation of the lower urinary tract.
- *Cystoscopic appearance:* The appearance of an invading mass can vary. A visible intra-luminal tumor may be easily seen or there may be distortion of the normal contour of the bladder due to mass effect.
- Patients should be managed by a multidisciplinary team. Extirpative procedures for persistent disease status post neoadjuvant therapy will typically require pelvic exenteration surgery.

Additional References for Consideration
- Management of Nonurological Pelvic Tumors Infiltrating the Lower Urinary Tract | SpringerLink.

References

1. Aldousari S, Kassouf W. Update on the management of non-muscle invasive bladder cancer. Cancer Urol Assoc J. 2010;4(1):56–64.
2. Donat M. Evaluation and follow-up strategies for superficial bladder cancer. Urol Clin North Am. 2003;30(4):765–76.
3. Zincke H, Ultz D, Farrow G. Review of Mayo Clinic experience with carcinoma in situ. Urology. 1985;26(4):39–46.
4. Nabi G, Greene D, O'Donnell MO. Suspicious urinary cytology with negative evaluation for malignancy in the diagnostic investigation of haematuria: how to follow up? J Clin Pathol. 2004;57(4):365–8.
5. Herr H. Role of repeat resection in non-muscle invasive bladder cancer. J Natl Compr Cancer Netw. 2015;13(8):1041–6.
6. Lamm D, Blumenstein B, Crissman J, et al. Maintenance bacillus Calmette-Guerin immunotherapy for recurrent Ta, T1 and carcinoma in situ TCC of the bladder: a randomized SWOG study. J Urol. 2000;163:1124–9.

7. Zabell J, Konety B. Management strategies for non-muscle-invasive bladder cancer (ta, T1, and CIS). In: Partin A, Dmochowski R, Kavoussi L, Peters C, editors. Campbell-Walsg-Wein. Philadelphia: Elsevier; 2021. p. 3091–111.

8. Pansadoro V, De Paula F. Intravesical bacillus Calmette-Guerin in the treatment of superficial transitional cell carcinoma of the bladder. J Urol. 1987;138(2):299–301.

9. Herr H, Dalbagani G. Defining bacillus Calmette-Guerin refractory superficial bladder tumors. J Urol. 2003;169(5):1706–8.

10. Shariat S, Palpattu G, Ameil G, et al. Characteristics and outcomes of patients with carcinoma in situ only at radical cystectomy. Urology. 2006;28(7):538–42.

11. Pernambuco-Holsten C. What Every Women Should Know about Bladder Cancer. Retrieved from Memorial Sloan Kettering Cancer Center: 2019. https://www.mskcc.org/news/what-every-woman-should-know-about-bladder.

12. Maxwell JP, Wang C, Wiebe N, Yilmaz A, Trpkov K. Long-term outcome of primary Papillary Urothelial Neoplasm of Low Malignant Potential (PUNLMP) including PUNLMP with inverted growth. Diagn Pathol. 2015;10:3.

13. Kates M, Bivalacqua T. Tumors of the bladder. In: Partin A, Dmochowski R, Kavoussi L, Peters C, editors. Campbell-Walsh-Wein urology. Philadelphia: Elsevier; 2021. p. 3073–90.

14. Guzzo T, Malkowicz B, Vaughn D, Wein A. Adult genitourinary cancer: prostate and bladder. In: Hanno P, Guzzo T, Malkowicz BW, editors. Penn clinical manual of urology. Philadelphia: Elsevier Inc; 2014. p. 505–8.

15. Amin MB, et al. Micropapillary variant of transitional cell carcinoma of the urinary bladder. Histologic pattern resembling ovarian papillary serous carcinoma. Am J Surg Pathol. 1994;18:1224–32.

16. Kamat AM, et al. Micropapillary bladder cancer. Cancer. 2007;110:62–7.

17. Mendelsohn G, Maksem JA. Divergent differentiation in neoplasms. Pathologic, biologic, and clinical considerations. Pathol Annu. 1986;21(1):91–119.

18. Shanks JH, Iczkowski KA. Divergent differentiation in urothelial carcinoma and other bladder cancer subtypes with selected mimics. Histopathology. 2009;54:885–900.

19. Mitra A, Bartsch C, Bartasch G, et al. Does presence of squamous and glandular differentiation in urothelial carcinoma of the bladder at cystectomy portend poor prognosis? An intensive case-control analysis. Urol Oncol. 2014;32:117–27.

20. Rausch S, Lotan Y, Youssef R. Squamous cell carcinogenesis and squamous cell carcinoma of the urinary bladder: a contemporary review with focus on nonbilharzial squamous cell carcinoma. Urol Oncol. 2014;32:11–32.

21. Steinberg GM. Bladder Cancer Staging. Retrieved from Medscape: 2020. http://emedicine.medscape.com

22. Vianella A, Costantini E, Del Zingaro M, et al. Repeated white-light transurethral resection of the bladder in nonmuscle invasive urothelial bladder cancers: systemic review and meta-analysis. J Endourol. 2011;25:1703–12.

23. Miladi M, Peyromaure M, Zerbib M, Saighi D, Debre B. The value of a second transurethral resection in evaluating patients with bladder tumours. Eur Urol. 2003;43(3):241–45.

24. Zabdell J, Badrinath K. Management strategies for non-muscle-invasive bladder cancer (ta, T1, and CIS). In: Partin A, Dmochowki R, Kavoussi L, Peters C, editors. Campbell-Walsh-Wein urology. Philadelphia: Elsevier; 2021. p. 3091–111.

25. Hurle R, Losa A, Manzetti A, Lembo A. Intravesical bacille Calmette-Guerin in stage T1 grade 3 bladder cancer therapy: a 7-year follow-up. Urology. 1999;54(2):258–63.

26. Chang S, Boorjian S, Chour R, et al. Diagnosis and treatment of non-muscle invasive bladder cancer: AUA/SUO joint guideline. J Urol. 2016;196:1021–9. Retrieved from American Urology Association

27. Tomio A, Kaiyo T. Clinicopathological and molecular characteristics of gastric and colorectal carcinomas in the elderly. Pathol Int. 2007;57(6):304–14.

28. Xiao PM, Bowne WM, Blank WM, Mason CM, Yang YM, Desoto FM, et al. Sigmoid colon cancer or urinary bladder cancer? Am J Gastroenterol. 2006:283–4.

29. Million RR, Fletcher G. Stage IV carcinoma of the cervic with bladder invasion. Am J Obst Gynecol. 1972;113:239–46.
30. Singh N, Hirschowitz L, Zaino R, al, e. Pathologic prognostic factors in endometrial carcinoma (other than tumor type and grade). Int J Gynecol Pathol. 2019;38(1):93–113.
31. American Cancer Society. *Survival Rates for Endometrial Cancer*. (2022). Retrieved from Cancer.org: https://www.cancer.org/cancer/endometrial-cancer/detection-diagnosis-staging/survival-rates.html#:~:text=5-year%20relative%20survival%20rates%20for%20endometrial%20cancer%20, All%20SEER%20stages%20combined%20%20%2081%25%20
32. Jemal A, Siegel R, Ward E, Murray T, Xu J, Thun M. Cancer statistics. CA: A Cancer J Clin. 2007;57:43–66.
33. Falch C, Amend B, Muller S, et al. Management of nonurological pelvic tumors infiltrating the lower urinary tract. Curr Surg Rep. 2014;2(11):1–11.
34. Kaur H, Verschraegen C. Cervical cancer. In: Silverman PM, editor. Oncologic imaging a Mult-displinary approach. Philadelphia: Elsevier; 2012. p. 441–53.
35. Nerli R, Ghagane S, Ram P, Shimikore S, Vinchurkar K, Hiremath M. Bladder invasion in patients with advanced colorectal carcinoma. Indian J Surg Oncol. 2018;9(4):547–51.
36. Strauss D, Hayes A, Thomas J. Retroperitoneal tumors: review of management. Ann R Coll Surg Engl. 2011;93:275–80.

Index